"'Do psychoanalysts have a story to tell?', asks Gregorio Kohon. Yes, he says, but not one that everybody wants to hear. Kohon presents psychoanalysis as a unique relationship between individuals that in principle can never be understood completely. He criticises attempts to tame psychoanalysis, making it more manageable by distorting its essential singularity. The book's wide-ranging discussion of these themes is enjoyably clear and direct. Kohon relates psychoanalysis to scientific, social and political ideologies, insisting on its true character in a way that is valuable in itself, and especially needed today."

– **Michael Parsons**, *British Psychoanalytical Society and French Psychoanalytic Association*

"Gregorio Kohon's book is a passionate, evocative and persuasive defence of the particular nature of the psychoanalytic endeavour. Kohon argues that, belonging neither to science nor to art, and yet to both, psychoanalysis is a unique and intimate encounter between two people that confronts the complexities of the human mind and in which fundamental primary phantasies can emerge in symptoms, dreams and the ever-evolving changes in the relationship itself. With this in mind, Kohon argues for the pre-eminence of the clinical case report as the most truly meaningful way in which the psychoanalytic method can be understood and its value assessed."

– **Priscilla Roth**, *Training Analyst and Fellow of the British Psychoanalytical Society*

"This powerful new book by Gregorio Kohon addresses the disquieting question of how we may best study and give credence to that singular endeavour, psychoanalysis. Kohon argues that psychoanalytic clinical practice and 'evidence based' research differ fundamentally in aim and approach. At the heart of his book lies the immense and irreducible complexity ('the unbridled imagination') of psychoanalysis, exemplified by two psychoanalytic case studies that give a real sense of the paradoxical and conjectural nature of the analytic couple at work. For Kohon, psychoanalysis itself is also the analyst's prime research tool."

– **Helen Taylor Robinson**, *Child Analyst and Fellow of the British Psychoanalytical Society*

Concerning the Nature of Psychoanalysis

In his new book, *Considering the Nature of Psychoanalysis: The Persistence of a Paradoxical Discourse*, Gregorio Kohon describes the complexity of the psychoanalytic encounter, questioning the misguided attempts to simplify and/or reduce it to either art or science.

Kohon disputes the contemporary use of parameters offered by evidence-based medicine as a research model to study psychoanalysis. Instead, he proposes to reconsider the relevance of the psychoanalytic single case study, its importance and pre-eminence.

The present book will be of great interest to all psychotherapists, councillors, psychiatrists, mental health workers and students and academics of the social sciences.

Gregorio Kohon is a Training Analyst of the British Psychoanalytical Society. Among other books, he edited *The Dead Mother: The Work of André Green* (1999) and *British Psychoanalysis: New Perspectives on the Independent Tradition* (2018). He also published *Love and its Vicissitudes* (co-authored with André Green, 2005) and *Reflections on the Aesthetic Experience: Psychoanalysis and the Uncanny* (2016).

THE NEW LIBRARY OF PSYCHOANALYSIS
General Editor: Alessandra Lemma

The New Library of Psychoanalysis was launched in 1987 in association with the Institute of Psychoanalysis, London. It took over from the International Psychoanalytical Library which published many of the early translations of the works of Freud and the writings of most of the leading British and Continental psychoanalysts.

The purpose of the New Library of Psychoanalysis is to facilitate a greater and more widespread appreciation of psychoanalysis and to provide a forum for increasing mutual understanding between psychoanalysts and those working in other disciplines such as the social sciences, medicine, philosophy, history, linguistics, literature and the arts. It aims to represent different trends both in British psychoanalysis and in psychoanalysis generally. The New Library of Psychoanalysis is well placed to make available to the English-speaking world psychoanalytic writings from other European countries and to increase the interchange of ideas between British and American psychoanalysts. Through the *Teaching Series*, the New Library of Psychoanalysis now also publishes books that provide comprehensive, yet accessible, overviews of selected subject areas aimed at those studying psychoanalysis and related fields such as the social sciences, philosophy, literature and the arts.

The Institute, together with the British Psychoanalytical Society, runs a low-fee psychoanalytic clinic, organizes lectures and scientific events concerned with psychoanalysis and publishes the *International Journal of Psychoanalysis*. It runs a training course in psychoanalysis which leads to membership of the International Psychoanalytical Association – the body which preserves internationally agreed standards of training, of professional entry, and of professional ethics and practice for psychoanalysis as initiated and developed by Sigmund Freud. Distinguished members of the Institute have included Michael Balint, Wilfred Bion, Ronald Fairbairn, Anna Freud, Ernest Jones, Melanie Klein, John Rickman and Donald Winnicott.

Previous general editors have included David Tuckett, who played a very active role in the establishment of the New Library. He was followed as general editor by Elizabeth Bott Spillius, who was in turn followed by Susan Budd and then by Dana Birksted-Breen. Current members of the Advisory Board include Giovanna Di Ceglie, Liz Allison, Anne Patterson, Josh Cohen and Daniel Pick.

Previous members of the Advisory Board include Christopher Bollas, Ronald Britton, Catalina Bronstein, Donald Campbell, Rosemary Davies, Sara Flanders, Stephen Grosz, John Keene, Eglé Laufer, Alessandra Lemma, Juliet Mitchell, Michael Parsons, Rosine Jozef Perelberg, Richard Rusbridger, Mary Target and David Taylor.

For a full list of all the titles in the New Library of Psychoanalysis main series as well as both the New Library of Psychoanalysis 'Teaching' and 'Beyond the Couch' subseries, please visit the Routledge website.

THE NEW LIBRARY OF PSYCHOANALYSIS

General Editor: Alessandra Lemma

Concerning the Nature of Psychoanalysis

The Persistence of a Paradoxical Discourse

Gregorio Kohon

Routledge
Taylor & Francis Group
LONDON AND NEW YORK

First published 2019
by Routledge
2 Park Square, Milton Park, Abingdon, Oxon OX14 4RN

and by Routledge
52 Vanderbilt Avenue, New York, NY 10017

Routledge is an imprint of the Taylor & Francis Group, an informa business

British Library Cataloguing-in-Publication Data
A catalogue record for this book is available from the British Library

Library of Congress Cataloging-in-Publication Data
A catalog record has been requested for this book

ISBN: 978-0-367-23650-2 (hbk)
ISBN: 978-0-367-23651-9 (pbk)
ISBN: 978-0-429-28102-0 (ebk)

Typeset in Bembo
by Swales & Willis, Exeter, Devon, UK

Contents

Acknowledgements

I am grateful to Professor David Leon for introducing me to the *Cochrane Database of Systematic Reviews* (*CDSR*), with its usefulness and the complexity of the data supplied by it (personal communication, 2012). I am also grateful to Dr Silvana I. L. Kohon, who helped me to clarify further the subtleties concerning the implementation by GPs of the relevant information given by the *CDSR* (personal communication, 2018).

My thanks to Alessandra Lemma, as Editor of the New Library of Psychoanalysis, and to Kate Hawes, from Routledge, for their support for my work. Also, my thanks to Eric and Klara King, for their help with the editing of the different versions of the present text.

I would like to thank Taylor and Francis, LLC, for permission to reprint the case of "Tony" (Chapter 2), published in an earlier version as "Love in a time of madness", in A. Green & G. Kohon, *Love and Its Vicissitudes* (London: Routledge, 2005), pp. 41–100. My gratitude to the following publications for the use of the case of "Barbara" (Chapter 3), which was included, in different versions, in the following journals: *Psicoanalisi – Rivista della Asociazone Italiana di Psicoanalisis,* for "Amore nel transfert. Identificazione primaria e imago materna (*14*, #2, July–Dec. 2010, pp. 2–20); *Revista de Psicoanálisis de la Asociación Psicoanalítica de Madrid,* for "Amor en transferencia. Identificación primaria e imago materna" (2012, *66*, pp. 119–136), and *Le présent de la psychanalyse, Association Psychanalytique de France,* for "Scènes de meurtre" (Jan. 2019, *1*, pp. 43–63).

All efforts have been made to obtain the necessary copyrights. Any omission in the present edition will be corrected in future.

I would like to express my special gratitude to Toni Griffiths for the continuing dialogue over things that matter.

My gratitude to Valli Shaio Kohon for her permission to use her *Wholly and in Part* … (2015) for the cover image.

Preface

Much has been written in recent decades about both critical social theory and psychoanalysis. Such writings have addressed the question of human subjectivity and the development of the self as well as the intricate, difficult, complex connections between these phenomena and social processes. Many authors have attempted, in different ways and from different points of view, to construct, develop, and critically evaluate theories that concern the place of the subject within modern culture. They have described in contemporary ideologies the prevalence of political values imposed by the affluent consumerist society, the corresponding commodification of culture, the apathy of the individual towards social commitment, and the consequent crises and breakdown of the ethical foundations of social concern.

In the beginning, the relation of the individual's unconscious to history and social change formed part of Freud's theoretical speculations. It also provoked intense debate among his followers: if the Freudian mind had a history, was the unconscious capable of change through the external historical changes occurring in society? Could a change in the structure of the modern family, for example, affect the unconscious dynamics of the Oedipus complex? Since, as Richard Wollheim has written, "We are born sexual but we are not born moral" (1984, p. 199), how does the culture in which we live contribute to the emergence of the individual's morality, which ultimately inspires and directs behaviour?

The concept of *ideology* can tentatively be characterised as the prevalent social meanings created, developed, and imposed by a given group, institution, or society through their ideals, principles, doctrines, myths, laws, and so on. Without expanding here on how ideology comes into being, one of its functions serves to impose and perpetuate dominance through masking or illusion, thus becoming a true barrier to social justice and change (Haslanger, 2017).

Reflecting in this context on the nature of psychoanalysis, how do conflicts between the prevalent ideology of a certain culture and the individual's own ideals operate in contemporary psychoanalysis? What are the ideals that, at present, affect psychoanalysts? Have the ideological and cultural changes in our society influenced us and determined changes in our psychoanalytic views? In our methods? In our approaches?

Psychoanalysts are compelled to concern themselves with these questions, but this does not mean that they are in a privileged position to give account of sociological and political problems.

Over a long period throughout the last century, psychoanalysts and their findings made important contributions in the UK and the rest of the world, not just within the mental health professions, but also in related fields like social work, education, general practice and paediatrics, and institutional functioning. Now, as a consequence of profound and, in effect, reactionary ideological changes in the policies of governments, professionals in the health and public services have been commanded to justify their practices.

Such a demand can be made to appear reasonable enough. Michael Rustin has written that

> when the taxpayer is paying, it is not enough that individuals find the services useful, or that professionals within the services do so. "Evidence of effectiveness" is expected... .
>
> (Rustin, 2001, p. 82)

From a different point of view, Felicitas Rost, President of the Society for Psychotherapy Research, argued that "psychoanalysis ... has a social responsibility in respect to providing *evidence of the effectiveness* of its treatment models" (2018, p. 8; italics added).

This presents a critical and problematic challenge: "evidence of effectiveness" through empirically demonstrable results is not easily achieved in psychoanalysis. This book aims to show why – at least, in part – that is so. The book is fundamentally concerned with the nature of psychoanalysis in its very specific sense: the individual treatment of single cases.

As part of this concern it also explores the shortcomings of certain types of research that aim to preserve a psychoanalytic presence in the public health sector. I do not, of course, object to these interventions; on the contrary, I am sympathetic to those psychoanalytically inspired professionals wishing to work, participate, and contribute in this area. In my 48 years of practice as a clinician, I have participated at times in different countries and in various professional capacities in the public sector.

My concern here is different. In response to the demands for simplified results concerning the efficacy of therapeutic treatments in general, a risk has emerged of an equally deficient response concerning both the theory and practice of psychoanalysis. In the last decade or so there has been a persistent, increasingly intense, and often misguided shift in some sectors of psychoanalytic psychotherapy and psychoanalysis, representing a move towards a highly reductive concept of scientific research which constitutes itself as an ideal, measuring the outcomes of therapeutic intervention in ways that neglect the very nature of psychoanalysis. As a consequence, it has devalued the central importance and significance of the single case study.

Are we being "forced" in certain areas to conform to political ideals that are not in tune with the aims and methods of psychoanalysis, either in our institutional participation or in our individual consulting rooms? Accountability is confused with measuring the outcomes of therapeutic intervention. In both cases, in misunderstanding and devaluing the central importance of the single case study, the very nature of psychoanalysis is neglected.

Chapter 1 argues that psychoanalysis is neither a science nor an art but inhabits a place of its own, with its necessary characteristics and approaches; it cannot be defined by, nor can it be assessed on, the terms and parameters of other disciplines. It is the study of single cases that has pushed psychoanalytic theory and practice forward; psychoanalysis is learnt through the studies of *exemplars* (Thomas Kuhn's concept) – single clinical cases.

Chapter 2 describes the lengthy analytic treatment of "Tony" – a psychotic young man, once described by a hospital psychiatrist as paranoid schizophrenic, trapped in a difficult relationship with his mother, struggling to survive between the fear of madness and the need to be mad. Working with him offered me the opportunity to treat somebody who, while being seriously disturbed and for a considerable time psychotic, was able to respond to psychoanalytic treatment.

Chapter 3 represents a different clinical presentation. The case of "Barbara" is presented, a woman unable to have close relationships, always feeling unsafe, inevitably threatened by an identification with a dangerous maternal imago. This primary imago, on the one hand, epitomised an omnipotent, protective, and sacred figure, a benign presence that could justifiably be described as "maternal". And yet, on the other hand, the same imago revealed a vulnerable and yet persecuting, pathetic figure dominated by helplessness, sadness, illnesses, and inhibitions.

Chapter 4 further develops the reflections on the two cases presented in the previous chapters. When the subjects in analysis are capable of accepting the existence of a psychic reality alien to themselves, when they recognise that their self contains something secret or different or contradictory to their wishes and thoughts, and that this something might be part of a conflict that is making them suffer, we say that they are psychologically minded. While Tony could contemplate the idea that anything that took place in the psychic scenario of his mind had a meaning and thus was worth thinking about, Barbara could not fully comprehend, nor did she wish to understand, the disturbance of her psychic internal world.

Chapter 5 puts forward the idea (following André Green's suggestions) of a "normal" madness, which is different from psychosis: it is not an occasional alteration in adult mental life. Instead, it is an inevitable component of psychic life throughout the subject's life – as long as the subject continues to experience emotions and is capable of passion. It is first experienced in the initial encounter with mother, and it will be at the core of the subject's unconscious. Subjectivity and relative neurotic normality appear as genuinely heroic achievements.

Chapter 6 addresses the question of the uncertainty of the psychoanalytic cure. As an object of research, it is inherently limited, and it remains an enormous challenge. In this context, how can the psychoanalyst accurately describe the logic of the unconscious, where reasons and causes, pain and pleasure, past and present are inevitably entangled and implicated? In reviewing the literature, it would appear that the evidence-based movement in psychotherapy may not provide a sufficiently meaningful basis for the evidence that is so strongly desired.

Chapter 7 proposes that psychoanalysis works through abductive inference, where hypotheses are put forward as questions. Being a subjective discipline, objectivity in psychoanalysis is neither attainable nor desirable; although there is a potential for a multiplicity of interpretations, there is only one experience, "that … which the analyst … had with his patient" (Bion, 1994, p. 7). It is up to the individual psychoanalyst to legitimise that experience.

1

PSYCHOANALYSIS

A literature of excess

Psychoanalysis constitutes a body of knowledge, acquired and developed through study and personal experience, the object of which is the psychic reality of the human subject. Psychic reality, as understood in psychoanalysis, cannot be reduced to either the mental or the physical, for the psychoanalytic object is neither exclusively psycho nor soma; it has its own characteristics, categories and laws (Gomez, 2005). Psychoanalytic models and theories are based on fundamental hypotheses and basic assumptions that have been arrived at through a mixture of clinical experience and self-reflection, speculative intellectual activity and intuition, free-floating attention and deduction, and the attribution of retrospective meaning and abstract representations.

Are we to regard psychoanalysis as a scientific discipline? What do we understand by the concept of science in the first place? Or should we just speak of psychoanalysis in terms of an art (Ogden, 2005)? Or something else?

Psychoanalytic theory oversteps the limits of moderation; it possesses an exuberance of creativity (Kohon, 1999, p. 149). It is a literature of excess that describes the existence and persistence of incestuous wishes, speaks in terms of life and death, and deals with uncontrollable passions and the potential presence of murderous feelings towards our loved ones; it attempts to give account of unconscious phantasies and demonstrates that what sometimes appear as "good intentions" can be the disguised expression of destructive envy. It has amply shown the inevitable splitting of the ego, the negation of what consciously we know, the existence of infantile sexual theories that continue to influence our adult psychic life – and much else.

I have previously argued that

> Since the unconscious cannot be domesticated, there is no possibility for the development of a psychoanalytic theory that would be definitive and unitary; as a theory, psychoanalysis is a deconstructing method which never reaches an absolute conclusion. Psychoanalysis can be understood as an attempt to develop an objective knowledge of subjectivity, but this act of knowledge is always under the inevitable influence of the subject's unconscious.
> (Kohon, 1999, p. 150)

Since its inception, there have been serious and critical misunderstandings concerning the nature of this strange discipline, some of them created and promoted by its own practitioners. Freud, in a letter to Fliess, declared,

> I am actually not at all a man of science, not an observer, not an experimenter, not a thinker. I am by temperament nothing but … an adventurer … with all the curiosity, daring, and tenacity characteristic of a man of this sort.
> (Freud, 1900, p. 398)

And yet, in wanting his creation to be accepted by society, Freud was the first to be responsible for the misplaced ideals of scientism that have contaminated the idea of a psychoanalytic discipline to this day. Despite Freud's own contradictions, the attacks on his personal integrity and professional honesty, and "whatever the simplification, abstruse spurious logic and downright falsification … " of his theoretical ideas (Grubrich-Simitis, 1995, p. 1), the real strength of Freudian psychoanalysis continues to reside in its insistence and tenacity, in its commitment to the remarkable persistence of its paradoxical discourse.

Cornelius Castoriadis remarked that human beings are not characterised by logic and rationality but by a radical, "unbridled imagination", which exercises a central role in our psyche, distinguishing us from the rest of the animal world (1988). Primates may be able to suck their thumbs, but they have not yet created language, music, science, literature, psychoanalysis, and art. Psychoanalysis owes its existence to, and continues to be developed by, this unbridled imagination in the "other scene" of an unconscious that Freud managed first to identify, to recognise, and to study.

Psychoanalysis finds its purpose in the therapeutic process that takes place in the exclusivity of the consulting-room, where patient and analyst gain access to the patient's unconscious in an encounter through language, marked by the dynamics of transference and countertransference. In dealing with neurosis, psychosis and other pathological presentations, psychoanalysts do not consider them as things in themselves: their symptoms always signify something else, something other.

Since the psychic processes under scrutiny are unconscious, there is no tangible or measurable method that offers any evidence for the accuracy of hypotheses and assumptions, other than what is offered from within the psychoanalytic method and setting. This does not necessarily render psychoanalysis inadequate nor ineffective: rather, it confronts the fact that "truth" is not an absolute concept, and thus it cannot be fully established. Within the realm of psychoanalytic clinical thought, theories become validated when the individual subject in analysis makes her own the interpretations offered by the analyst. Every interpretation is tried and tested, as it were, in every new situation in which it appears; it is then that theoretical ideas become personal knowledge.

I referred above to "misplaced ideals of scientism". Psychoanalysis is neither a science nor an art but inhabits a place of its own, with its necessary characteristics and approaches. At the same time, there are experiences encountered in the many and different quests for understanding and meaning across different disciplines which link considerations in psychoanalysis to considerations within other disciplines (and vice versa). This is obviously not to say that psychoanalysis should be defined and assessed within the terms of another discipline.

I illustrate these points by reference to four ideas which have interdisciplinary meaning and resonance: *indeterminancy, undecidability, over-determination*, and *hypercomplexity*.

1. *Indeterminancy*. One of the fundamental discoveries of quantum mechanics has led to the principle of indeterminacy. Rovelli argues that

> it is not possible to predict exactly ... where an electron will appear tomorrow. Between one appearance and another, the

> electron has no precise position, as if dispersed in a cloud of probability ... Spacetime is a physical object like an electron. It, too, can be in a 'superposition' of different configurations.
>
> (Rovelli, 2017, pp. 75–79)

Superposition, fluctuation, blurring, indetermination – this is the language of the physicists: "'Fluctuation' does not mean that what happens is never determined. It means that it is determined only at certain moments, and in an unpredictable way" (Rovelli, 2017, p. 77).

This indeterminacy, a concept describing something that cannot be clearly defined or completely known, applies to the object of psychoanalytic study, to the knowledge arrived at through psychoanalytic enquiry and to the therapeutic implications derived from it.

Psychoanalysis can be compared to how music was conceived by John Cage, the American composer who created the indeterminacy movement in New York in the 1950s. Cage originally defined indeterminacy as "the ability of a piece to be performed in substantially different ways" (Pritchett, 1993, p. 108). In psychoanalysis, the choice of each interpretation given to a patient is determined by a multiplicity of factors. Nevertheless, the act of giving the interpretation can be compared to the performance of a musical composition that is not clearly noted or precisely specified beforehand; in the best clinical moments in the consulting-room, there is also an "indeterminacy of performance" (Simms, 1986, p. 357). According to Cage, the only true form of indeterminate music is when chance elements intervene in the very moment of performance. Obviously, a psychoanalytic interpretation is not chosen by chance, but the analyst does not have a written, analytic "score". There is no sheet music, as it were, no prior representation of the interpretation, no pre-published, noted text. Analysts have to follow their own gut feelings; interpretations will come from a mixture of instinctive emotional responses, creative imagination, and the capacity to identify with the other and from the analyst's own intellectual courage.

2. *Undecidability*. This concept originates in the specific nature of computability theory and computational complexity theory: an undecidable problem is a decision problem to which it is impossible to construct a single algorithm leading to a correct answer, whether negative or positive. This is closely linked to the questions

originally posed by Gödel's theorems (1931), where a statement is neither provable nor refutable within a specified deductive system. The undecidability of a statement in a particular deductive system does not, in and of itself, address the question of whether the truth value of the statement is well-defined or whether it can be determined by other means; undecidability only indicates that the particular deductive system being considered cannot prove the truth or falsity of the statement. Gödel showed that it is impossible to be completely truthful and completely universal; you can never say a true statement without saying some false ones. Alternatively, you can never say only true things without being forced to withhold some other equally true statements (Berto, 2009).

In psychoanalysis, there are only "absolutely undecidable" interpretative constructions: their value cannot be fully known – they are only theory, not "discoveries" in the conventional sense. For the psychoanalyst, however, they help to make visible what is not comprehensible or understandable. More than anything else, and much more importantly, they develop the conditions through which psychoanalytic theory organises itself so that the unconscious of the other, as expressed in the clinic, can be revealed. Castoriadis (1997) believed that one of the best examples of how our imagination creates theoretical structures in which the psychic may be thought is Freud's "Project" (1959 [1895]), his unfinished work where he created an imaginary constructum through his capacity to reflect and to think. We may need, therefore, to imagine our psychic world in order to be able to think anything about it. To imagine, to phantasise, to create new ways of thinking ... This form of proceeding might not be that distant nor alien to traditional science. According to Rovelli, "The ability to understand something *before* it's observed is at the heart of scientific thinking" (2017, p. 10).

3. *Over-determination.* This concept, introduced by Freud in *Studies on Hysteria* (1895), concerns something that operates at all levels of human life. For example, geneticists have long known that it is always the interaction of a variety of genes interacting with internal and external environmental factors that determines biologically important consequences – big and small: "Genes do not operate in a vacuum, but, rather, each has its role to play in the complex machinery of development" (Neel & Schull, 1954, p. 27).

In psychoanalysis, the notion of over-determination helps us to describe the many and diverse formations of the unconscious.

Whether a dream or a symptom, a particular formation is never the result of one cause alone. A formation is always "related to a multiplicity of unconscious elements which may be organised in different meaningful sequences, each having its own specific coherence at a particular level of interpretation" (Laplanche & Pontalis, 1967, p. 292).

4. *Hypercomplexity*. The epistemological concept of *hypercomplexity*, developed in the contemporary sciences, confirmed the idea of a totalising or unitary knowledge as an illusion. We are witnessing a displacement of epistemological questions by ontological realities in sciences like biology, where scientists find it difficult to describe different levels of complexity in cells and in systems. Such systems represent complex configurations of parts, factors, and forces that interact with each other. At times, a particular event or fact is the result of diverse direct or indirect non-linear feedback sequences. In trying to study this hypercomplexity, biologists find it difficult to think of models that are adequate to describe those systems. In these circumstances, scientists might find themselves predicting responses without being able to explain the properties of the systems causing the response.[1]

The concept of hypercomplexity is also used in the social sciences. For Qvortrup (1998), this notion defines a second-order complexity, *a complexity inscribed in complexity*, which has emerged as a new social paradigm in contemporary society. Qvortrup did not attempt to describe the hypercomplexity of society in his work; instead, he used the concept as an explanatory category applied to the observation of certain specific processes in society. Qvortrup argued that hypercomplexity refers to a dominant social semantics governing the understanding of society and characterised by polycentrism. In other words, there is no one single and universal position from which to observe social phenomena; rather, there are many observation points, each of them using an individual observational code specific to its own social complexity. In astronomy, the parallax or peripatetic view refers to the apparent position of a star among more distant stars, a position that changes when viewed from opposite sides of the earth's orbit. In general physics, it refers to an apparent change in the position of an object resulting from a change in the observer's position (see Kohon, 2016, pp. 87–88). Furthermore, many observations are observations of observations, making them not only polycentric but also polycontextual.

Indeterminacy, undecidability, over-determination, hypercomplexity: these are but some illustrations of the complexity of the quest for knowledge and understanding in different fields. In psychoanalysis, how do we find and establish adequate parameters that correspond to, and would give proper account of, the complexity of human subjects and the diversity of their psychic life? It is not so much a matter of how to know the reality of what the research intends to investigate but, rather, what that reality is.

As early as in 1893, Freud declared,

> … it still strikes me myself as strange that the case histories I write should read like short stories and that, as one might say, they lack the serious stamp of science. I must console myself with the reflection that *the nature of the subject is evidently responsible for this*, rather than any preference of my own.
>
> (Freud, 1893, p. 159, italics added)

Ontological questions must necessarily precede epistemological ones (Scott & Usher, 1996; see also Žižek, 1998).

In the psychoanalytic tradition, this formidable and yet problematic challenge has been approached through the detailed study of single clinical cases. Psychoanalytic case studies originated in clinical medicine, traditionally representing an in-depth investigation, over an extended period of time, of a single person: the case history, the patient's personal history. However, in psychoanalysis, in contrast to medicine, data are not gathered using several different methods, from a variety of sources.

The clinical case study in psychoanalysis consists of a written description of a treatment, characterised as an idiographic approach,[2] emphasising the unique personal experience of a subject. Perelberg describes, for example, how in Freud's clinical presentations there is a simultaneous study of structure and history. In each of his clinical cases, says Perelberg, " … Freud constructed hypotheses about the successive stages that gave rise to the structure" (Perelberg, 2005, p. 14): *hypotheses*, then, *constructed* by the psychoanalyst. Such study does not seek to formulate laws nor generalise results that are *necessarily* applicable to other subjects; whatever the hypothesis and/or conclusions, there is neither assumption nor certainty that they would correspond to other cases.

As the earlier illustrations of complexity also suggest, outcome studies and empirical forms of research do not contribute new information to the discipline of psychoanalysis (see Chapter 6, herein). The aims of empirical researchers, as valuable as their studies may be, are different to those of psychoanalysts who write up their cases, attempting to share their clinical experience with colleagues, communicating their own personal and professional findings. If there are new psychoanalytic breakthroughs, whether theoretical or therapeutic, they emerge from the work carried out by the individual psychoanalyst in the consulting room with the patient.

Perception of events depends on how the percipient conceives the world: two observers witnessing the same phenomenon may be steeped in two radically different theories and thus will see two different things. Such methodological incommensurability, a concept central to psychoanalysis, excludes any universal mode of making inferences from the observed. Furthermore, the observed itself is changed by the observer; there is no possibility of making references to a fixed, permanent goal (Kuhn, 1962, p. 173).

A psychoanalytic case study takes into consideration not only the patient's subjectivity but also that of the psychoanalyst. The effectiveness of psychoanalytic interventions is assessed by the movement of the analytic process itself, by the changes from session to session as well as within one single session. The analyst registers these movements by paying special attention to the dynamics of transference and countertransference and to the responses of the analysand to interpretations: that is, have they produced new, meaningful information? Have new memories been uncovered? Is the process of free association being helped by the analyst's intervention? Is the patient's narrative creating new meanings? Can some of patient's responses be indicative of psychic change?

In spite of their difficulties and limitations, case studies have been the very type of study which has pushed psychoanalytic theory forward. And yet, by definition, the psychoanalytic clinical case possesses, like all great works of literature (including Freud's writings), the "uncanny ability to evolve endlessly diverse readings" (Bloom, 1986, p. 26). It never yields "scientific" generalisations. Indeed, at times, the achievements reached by psychoanalysis in the consulting-room may be rather modest. For example, psychoanalysts would consider it to be progress whenever the patient on the couch responds to the analyst's interpretation by saying, "that makes me think of … ", followed by a genuine, free association (André Green, quoted in Caldwell, 1995; see also Browne & Streeruwitz, 2017, p. xxv).

This is not what is commonly thought to constitute "scientific" evidence – but it *is* psychoanalysis.

There is another kind of methodological rigour, described by Pontalis (2000) as poetic – that is, creative, in the sense of the original Greek word, *poetikós*. Instead of lacking precision, the poetic rigour of psychoanalysis represents a concern for the right word, uttered at the right moment. Pontalis argues that,

> In this respect, it is faithful to dreams: a dream is never vague in the choice of images that it employs to express the message it carries - it couldn't be more exact … Dreams, poetry, analysis: the exact sciences.
>
> (Pontalis, 2000, p. 76)

Carlo Rovelli, the renowned theoretical physicist, Director of the Quantum Gravity Research Group at the *Centre de physique théorique* in Marseille, France, also argues that, "Perhaps poetry is another of the deepest roots of science: the capacity to see beyond the visible" (Rovelli, 2017, p. 21, translation modified). Another kind of "commonality of experience" (see Kohon, 2016, p. 19)?

Thomas Kuhn's *The Structure of Scientific Revolutions* (1962), in which he expounded his views of revolutionary scientific changes, represented a historical landmark in the philosophy of science. Years later, he presented a paper entitled, "What Are Scientific Revolutions?", in which he restated them, arguing that,

> Revolutionary change is defined in part by its difference from normal change … [which] results in growth, accretion, cumulative addition to what was known before ["normal process"]. … Revolutionary changes are different and far more problematic. They involve discoveries that cannot be accommodated within the concepts in use before they were made. In order to make or to assimilate such a discovery one must alter the way one thinks …
>
> (Kuhn, 1987, pp. 13, 32)

The evolution of scientific theory does not emerge from the straightforward accumulation of facts, a positivist view of science, but, rather, from a set of changing intellectual circumstances and possibilities. Revolutionary changes are not necessarily "rationally reconstructible" (Patton, 2014, p. 21); there is a need for new concepts and theoretical frameworks, new ways of thinking about and describing phenomena. Kuhn's concept of a shift in paradigm described a difference in the way that we experience and perceive things, a change in one's phenomenal world; the world changes as a result of the creation of a new paradigm (Hoyningen-Huene, 1990).

At the same time, Kuhn suggested another, different view, according to which the referent, the actual thing referred to by a concept, is determined through its similarity to a set of exemplary cases rather than by the signified, the meaning, the concept or idea that the sign expresses or evokes (Forrester, 2017b). This unorthodox understanding, Kuhn's change from *paradigms* to *exemplars*, offered an important alternative, the representation of the singular becoming a genuine, authentic possibility. Students of psychoanalysis learn through the exemplars of single clinical cases, through the problems and challenges presented by them and the possible responses to those problems. People wanting to train in psychoanalysis will be expected to know the psychoanalytic exemplars, from Freud's original clinical cases onwards. And there is, of course, no fixed set, no limited numbers of exemplars.[3]

Following his rendering and interpretation of Kuhn's ideas, Forrester proposes "reasoning in cases" (2017a). This sounds right: *reasoning in cases, thinking through cases.* Always to be borne in mind, however, is that the analyst is not there to tell the "full story" of a psychoanalytic treatment, nor could a completely accurate picture of a patient's predicament and/or pathology be created.

I present, in the following chapters, two contrasting clinical cases. My hope is to bring these different treatments to life in the minds of the readers.

A psychoanalytic writer does not work by the rules of a scientific method based on terms of confirmation or falsification. In Forrester's words, a psychoanalyst does not write just "*about* psychoanalysis"; the writing itself is subject "to the same laws and processes as the psychoanalytic situation itself" (Forrester, 2017c, p. 65). And, as a writer, one would want to be capable of "*infect(ing)* readers with the terms and frame of reference of the patient's analysis" (p. 86).

Infectious, that is, compelling, catching, or perhaps, more simply, *communicable*.

Notes

1 In algebra, for example, contemporary mathematicians speak of hypercomplex numbers, extensions of the complex numbers constructed by means of abstract algebra, such as quaternions and octonions (Kantor, Solodovnikov & Shenitzer, 1989). These extensions play an important role in a wide range of mathematical disciplines – for example, for the calculation of orbital mechanics of space vehicles and for computer vision development. To complicate matters further, mathematicians have described more than one type of hypercomplex number.

2 Idiographic, from the Greek word *idios*, means "own" or "private". The idiographic approach is radically opposed to the nomothetic view, which looks for universal laws of behaviour in order to be able to predict behaviour. In psychological studies, for example, personality is understood as consistent, largely inherited, and determined by genetics and biochemistry of the brain; in its extreme version, environmental factors, life's experiences, and social influences are not important factors to be considered.

3 In a different context, Tzvetan Todorov contrasts the dangers of "literal" memory with the acumen and awareness of "exemplary" memory. *Literal memory* would recall specific past events, retelling them over and over, as if to save them from oblivion; they are not examined in the context of a meaningful history and tend to be used instead as part of political agendas; they can tend to perpetuate, not only resentment but serve to fix categories of victims and perpetrators along prejudiced lines of race, ethnicity and national origin. *Exemplary memory* would revisit the past from a different perspective: not determined by the interests of any specific group but attempting instead to understand, without simplification or unchallenging explanations, what immoral, cruel, violent and/or grossly unfair historical behaviours and events can teach us about human nature and society (2000).

2

"TONY"

From the analysis of a psychotic young man

> There is only one illness: we are all ill *of* hate and *for* love.
> Enrique Pichon-Rivière (1965)

Although Tony could not trust his memory, he had always known that without memories he was nothing. He was aware that his past had been invented by his mother through a series of half-lies, illusions, and self-deceptions presented to herself and to the world as truths. He no longer fought with his mother about this; he knew that to argue with her was a fruitless, painful exercise. His mother was not necessarily aware of her capacity for conjuring up people and events from the past in a way that did not remotely reflect their reality. Tony knew that she was mad, but he was unable to put this into words until some time later in his analysis.

Tony's earliest memory was of a beer-garden in a country pub. He was playing on the swings with his sister while their mother and father drank, smoked, laughed, and talked to other people. He could remember sensations: the suffocating smell of tobacco on his mother's winter coat, his father's rather loud voice calling to a friend across the tables, his sister's graceful and dignified movements on the swing, his own fear of swings. He could remember an afternoon spent on the stony beaches of Brighton: he saw himself eating a big, long piece of the pink rock sold at sweet shops by the esplanade. He was sitting by the sea, feeling hot, unhappy, crying about something he could not account for, becoming afraid.

In fact, fear was what he remembered the most: fear of his father, fear of school, fear of the teachers, fear of the water, fear of the swings, fear of cars. These fears paralysed him. He could not swim, he hated travelling, the mere thought of an aeroplane made him throw up. He felt defeated by his lack of courage. When the children at school called him names, he imagined himself actually being transformed into a chicken, a rabbit, a rat. He would wake up at night sweating, shivering, seeing himself as a small animal floating on heavy seas, agitated and confused. He felt isolated. And yet it was these memories that gave him a sense of reassurance: after all, he was like anybody else, he had a family and a past. Life had some meaning.

The first time I saw Tony was in the context of a family interview with his mother and elder sister. He had been referred to a colleague who had invited me to participate as co-therapist. Tony was 21 years old; he had long hair, dirty clothes, and a smell that made one sick. It permeated everything. After he left the room, a truly offensive, noxious stench lingered in the air.

After a violent public outburst in a crowded street, he had been picked up by the police, who had to struggle to push him into one of their vans. Tony was diagnosed by the hospital psychiatrist as paranoid schizophrenic. He spent only three days in hospital, detained under the Mental Health Act; electroshock treatment had been strongly recommended, but his mother took him home after he begged her to support him in refusing treatment. She agreed. "I want to save my boy", she said to us. She offered to pay for one, perhaps two years of psychotherapy.

Tony had been "doing drugs" on a daily basis. I would later discover that at different times he had tried hashish and marijuana, mescaline, hallucinogenic mushrooms, and LSD. Given the culture of the time (early 1970s), this was not completely unexpected nor unusual; he had used these drugs occasionally, for recreational and experimental purposes only; he was not addicted. Tony's breakdown had taken place after a bad trip with LSD. He started feeling as if he were outside his body; he thought people were after him. He developed strange body sensations: a spot on his head, for example, grew into a big penis that was out of control. He felt that the pavement was pulsating, the trees breathing. He looked at himself in the mirror and turned into Paul McCartney. He screamed at a Leonard Cohen record cover, claiming that the singer had stolen his face. He shouted in the street that he wanted his soul back inside his body. He sat for long hours in the house where he was squatting with friends, thinking that everyone around him was dead. He had terrifying nightmares from which he found it difficult to wake.

In the family interview the mother did most of the talking, describing the family background and present circumstances. She dominated the scene and spoke on everybody's behalf. She was anxious, at times fairly manic; there was a histrionic side to her that made one feel part of the audience in a show. Tony's sister did not participate; clearly, she did not want to be there; she had her own life and her own problems to cope with. Tony said nothing and sat stiffly on his chair, looking lost. If asked anything, he responded mainly in mumbles and whispers. He kept his hands crossed over his stomach, as if holding himself in. From time to time, he would laugh, for no apparent reason. At the end of the family consultation, it was suggested that Tony come to see me in therapy. He glanced at me with a mixture of despair and defiance. It was the beginning of a therapeutic relationship that was to last 17 years.

Tony had grown up in a "typical" family in a Manchester suburb. Father, a businessman, had died from a heart attack when Tony was in his teens, shortly after the family had moved to London. Mother had been a teacher and was now retired. His only sister, 25 years old, left home at a young age to marry, but this did not last. While still living at home, she had spent a great deal of time complaining about their mother's preference for Tony. The mother had always spoken of him as her "prince". In fact, Tony had "believed" her story for many years: he was a real prince who had been given to her by the Royal Family. Of course, far from feeling great, as he was meant to, Tony felt weird, never comfortable in himself. Although he was very intelligent, he had not done well at school; always an outsider, he was unable to make many friends. He was perpetually teased by other kids and became excruciatingly self-conscious.

After his sister left home, Tony felt claustrophobic living with his mother. He was convinced that she wanted to have an incestuous relationship; he was terrified that she would get into bed with him at night; he felt utter disgust when she was near him and yet was afraid of having an erection if his mother physically approached him. All these feelings became unbearable, and he finally ran away from home. He lived as a squatter with other young people in a house owned by the then Greater London Council. He lived on unemployment benefits and, from time to time, accepted some financial help from his mother. Tony was quite musical, and for many years, while living as a dropout, he wanted to form a small rock'n'roll band. This was one of his few dreams, a project for the future …

During the first 18 months of treatment, a heavy and greatly charged silence dominated our meetings. Tony sat in front of me, eyes shut, saying nothing, maintaining an intense expression on his face. From time to time he mumbled a few words, or he would grumble and moan. Sometimes it was more a noise than a word that would come out of his mouth. The sessions left me in a dispirited and troubled mood; his misery made me feel hopeless. My efforts to establish a dialogue were mostly met with a silent, stony wall. Tony seemed to be living in a truly borderline state where the limits between his own self and the outer world were blurred. He was also in a hallucinatory state; the only way for him to maintain a certain sense of reality was to keep himself and the world immobile. To think something was to make it reality; all "bad" thoughts were terribly dangerous: murder and incest, homosexuality and madness were all too close to becoming realised. To talk about them, to pronounce these words, was equivalent to turning them into realities. Thus, Tony kept silent.

Life was a burden, libidinal drives were just too complicated; desires became persecutory. They evoked open landscapes full of dangers; they made Tony feel at sea; he wanted rigid walls around himself to feel safe. To the outside world he appeared "dead", as if living in an empty world. Concurrently, however, he established a very passionate, immediate, positive transference relationship with me, which was shown at the beginning, for example, by an intense reaction to arriving late for his sessions. On those occasions he became very upset, beside himself with anger and frustration. Tony had to travel far to get to my consulting room. He depended on the vicissitudes of public transport and had to combine catching buses with the underground; he had to time his journey very carefully. Nevertheless, Tony was unable to express the frustration or the anger he experienced through being late. If I made a reference to his rage, he took it as a suggestion to put his murderous feelings into action; he reacted with great anxiety and became confused. The same would apply to his feelings of attachment to me in the therapy, which, if interpreted, became the equivalent of a homosexual seduction. At other times, interpretations created a kind of short circuit in his mind; he refused to hear what I had to say, believing that I wanted to force my way into him. Tony experienced my interpretations as "doing" something to him; he could easily feel invaded by them, in which case he felt that I was poisoning him, or that he was taken over, like a flood of good milk that drowned him.

As reported by authors who have analysed psychotic patients, Tony took my interpretations in a very concrete way. Hanna Segal has described the difficulties of schizophrenic patients in forming symbols or in using them; if one interprets castration anxiety, let us say, the interpretation itself may be experienced by the patient as an actual act of castration (Segal, 1950, 1957). However, in contrast to Segal's description, Tony did not seem to have difficulties with the formation of symbols, nor did he have a serious inhibition in using them. In his case, the confusion between reality and its symbolic representations appeared to have taken place in the area of the self; in other words, Tony's confusion in understanding my interpretations was a consequence of the loss of boundaries between self and others (cf. Rosenfeld, 1952).

Tony presented many characteristics found in schizophrenic patients. For example, his catatonic posture at the beginning of the analysis was dominated by the classically described hyperconsciousness of such patients, which makes all forms of introspection painfully focused. The pseudo-detachment offered by his physical rigidity gave Tony a peculiar sense of power, as if standing back from experience could make him feel that the whole world depended on him. He, and only he, wished to give existence to the world outside and to the objects that existed there. Concerned at times with the very existence of the world, there was no apparent room or time in his life to be involved with more mundane things: jobs, career, normal sadness, the burden of everyday life.

The difficulties presented by schizophrenic patients who cannot form or use symbols, as well as the problems presented by patients like Tony, who experience temporary or chronic loss of boundaries between self and others, should both be distinguished from patients whom I have previously described as symbolically impoverished. The latter also confuse what is symbol and what is action, although their sense of self is not as seriously disturbed, making it possible for them to function in the world. For example, they do not experience themselves as possessing a body and a mind with no boundaries; they might appear connected to reality and have fairly normal relationships. Nevertheless, they experience these relationships as a series of actions: one is permanently doing something to someone else, and vice versa. The symbolically impoverished patient feels hated by everybody, and this is at the core of the predicament; as a result, words addressed to such a patient might be interpreted as acts of hatred requiring a defensive, hating response. Misunderstanding the analyst's interpretations becomes the central difficulty in the analysis of symbolically impoverished patients. They are able to experience hate of others (or feel the others' hate) but suffer from an inability to love (Kohon, 1999).

While silence prevailed during the initial part of Tony's treatment, this did not mean that the sessions were empty. Tony was under the spell of a much-idealised, positive, perhaps even magical transference that was easily threatened by his paranoid anxieties. He made me sharply aware of how little it took for me, as his analyst, to become a dangerous and persecuting figure. I, too, found myself in a very intense relationship with him. For example, I lived in fear that he might do something destructive, either to himself or to others. I would feel – although I never acted on these or similar feelings – a sudden urge to ring him between sessions. I had dreams about him that showed my own hopelessness and despair in treating him. In one of these dreams, in which I thought he had killed somebody, Tony was asking me compellingly, "Do you pray? Do you pray for me?"

Possibly such thoughts and dreams reflected communications coming from Tony, but they did not make me feel invaded, nor did I mind having them. They were a benign form of projective identification.[1] What distinguishes this from a malignant form of projective identification is that, although one finds oneself playing a part in somebody else's fantasy, one does not necessarily feel controlled from within. In other words, these two different forms can be assessed by considering their effect on the recipient subject. In the malignant, pathological form, the recipient of the projection feels the need to push the feelings back where they came from – that is, the feelings projected by the subject are felt as unwelcome by the other. In the benign form, the other person can contain the induced feelings without experiencing loss of freedom. This is similar to the distinction made by Bion between normal and abnormal psychotic projective identification, which is based on the degree of violence of the splitting, the force of the intrusion into the object, and the intensity of the hatred directed at it (Bion, 1959, 1962a). A malignant projective identification, for example, might not necessarily be solely used for defensive purposes; it could be used as a way of communicating unbearable experiences to the object (Rosenfeld, 1983). The character of projective identifications can also change value: what might be malignant at one stage can be processed, worked through, and turned into a benign form at another stage. During the process of analysis, under certain circumstances of severe stress, a benign form can also turn into a malignant, intrusive projective identification.

Occasionally, I used these experiences for my interpretations. I might suggest, for example, that Tony desperately wanted me to think about him over the weekend, that he wanted me to miss him as much as he missed me, that I should not allow any separation between us to exist. It was vital for Tony that I held him in my mind between sessions; it was something he himself was unable to do with me. On occasion, he was assailed by doubts about my existence and was tremendously relieved to see me at the next session. The omnipotent idealisation of his relationship with me, and his psychotic perception of me as his saviour and personal messiah, made it difficult for him to believe that I really existed – that I was not just a figment of his imagination.[2]

In psychosis, the confusion between love and hate, the extreme uncertainty about what is good and what is bad for the subject, also cause life and death to be confused. Tony had the omnipotent fantasy of "paralysing" time in order to eliminate the differences between being alive and being dead. In one session, he said, "I can't sleep next to Alice [his girlfriend], she feels too hot, I'll get burnt, I feel all cold inside me, my body doesn't exist, I can't shit, I can't fuck, I can't eat … to feel is like being torn to pieces, feelings are dangerous, I have nothing to say." On another occasion, he declared, "I want to retreat from life, to live is too dangerous for me, I'd like everything to be dead … when I walk down the streets, everything is still, like ice, I feel dead, I never left my mother's womb."

This confusion between birth and death seems to be particularly evident in most forms of psychotic thinking (Kohon, 1976). "Mr R", for example, had been a psychiatric patient for a while before coming to see me for treatment; he was living in a private therapeutic community while he attended analysis with me. On several occasions, he had to be hospitalised, and I visited him in hospital for his sessions. He was, despite his illness, incredibly resourceful but could not put this to good use. For example, Mr R once managed to get through several security checkpoints at the American Embassy – in the early 1970s, a truly ugly fortress in the middle of Mayfair. He was found in the consul's office, demanding to be given an explanation as to why he had been disqualified from going to Vietnam. On one occasion, Mr R came early to a session and locked himself in the toilet for a long while. This was not unusual, but when he lay down on the couch, he told me that he had tried to commit suicide in the toilet by drinking iodine from a bottle (which he had bought at the local chemist's on the way to the session). I was not sure whether to rush him to hospital immediately. Although he was coughing and his voice sounded rather hoarse, he did not seem very sick. I decided to wait. Then he announced, "I'm going to be reborn." Soon afterwards, I found out exactly what he meant: he defecated in his pants while lying on the couch – an event that was going to be repeated a couple of times during the treatment. In fact, Mr R had delusions of becoming a woman and giving birth to himself; he wanted to die so that he could come back as a woman; he wished to create himself once again. For him, to go to Vietnam was to have the likely chance of dying, so he would be sent back home in a coffin covered by an American flag; he would then be reunited with mother in glory and she would love him for ever. Mr R was caught in a deluded maintenance of a prenatal union with mother, never to be torn apart.

Mr R wanted to paralyse time. He lived a mummified existence; his actions were frozen acts without a morrow (Minkowski, 1933). The deliria of schizophrenic patients seems to be permanently crystallised in their fragmentation, forever running in the same place. This is reflected in schizophrenic coprophagy, in which there is a rejection of the irreversible character of physiological processes that conditions the irreversibility of biological temporality (Gabel, 1962). Mr R wanted to eat his excrement, just as Tony did. I never knew for sure whether he had ever done so. In the act of eating his own excrement, the subject denies having expelled it, denies even having had anything to expel. It is a model of what can be lost, and the attempt to re-incorporate the excrement is not only to recover it: it is the denial of the very possibility of losing it. Mr R also masturbated every day, compulsively; he claimed that he was able to suck his penis and swallow his own sperm. He commented once, "There is no waste this way …"

Tony had frequent visual, olfactory, and auditory hallucinations, which persisted, with varying intensities, over the first year of treatment. His visual hallucinations were usually connected to objects in the room: the telephone in the corner of my office became a nasty monkey, ready to pounce on him. Upon entering the room, he might have the experience of not recognising me. He would think he heard voices: somebody was whispering awful threats into his ear; he believed that the voices came through the opening in the fireplace or through the wall from the house next door. He insisted that I should feed him with the supposedly exotic food that he imagined somebody was cooking in the kitchen of my house.

Throughout these difficult times, I was encouraged by the fact that Tony did not act out in any major way. This was a source of great relief to me; it made the intensity and the frustration of my involvement with him bearable. Through his silence he was able to convey his gratitude. In not acting out, he was effectively looking after me and protecting our relationship.

In time, Tony proved to me that he did not lack words: in sharp contrast to the silence of the initial sessions, towards the end of the second year of analysis he began to write letters. This is part of the text of the first letter:

> *Dear Gregsie, Your fucking therapy is no good at all you cunt. It doesnt work … I want to kill people I mean kill someone I may kill someone literally take a fucking knife and stab some cunt … I want drugs LSD I want LSD now I want to go fucking crazy I need heroin I hurt … I no longer have any sexual desire thats not funny I want to kill women … Tie the fucking bitches up fuck'em in the arse and stab the cunts fuck their wounds and you too cunt you fucker … Im gonna fucking smash myself to bits I want to break myself up kill my fucking self … I just ate me dinner of the plate like a dog. So I'm back all full up and farting so I'm not angry anymore … What a cunt why do I have to come up there eh Why don't you come here. I don't want to earn any money … I'm a lot better now thanks doctor. Your office stinks of shit what sort of office is it a shite hole … This isn't*

> *funny ... I want 24hr recovery service my bodys all locked up ... A nice little explanation I want to be a star a fucking star I'm going to be a star.*[3]

Tony gave me this letter, scribbled on pages from a notebook, with an uncertain look on his face. I asked him whether he wanted me to read it there and then; he shrugged his shoulders. I decided to do so. He then asked me to keep it, and I agreed. Though I did not explicitly say this at the time, I considered his writing me a letter a step forward in our relationship; it was definite progress compared to communicating with me exclusively through projective identification. There was plenty of material for me to interpret, but initially, spontaneously, I only said, "It's tough luck you cannot be a fucking star." He looked at me, rather surprised; this encouraged me. I added a comment about his reference to the money: I said that I realised the uncertainty he was now facing, having to find funds to pay for his therapy. I said that he certainly would never get 24-hr recovery service, but that it would be a great loss if he could not even have the time of his sessions. He gave me a faint, painful smile. Then he broke down and burst into tears. For the rest of that session, we remained in silence.

In the following session, he produced another letter:

> *I don't care if I' conjuring up your presence. Wouldnt you? Schizophrenia isn't all laughs. There comes a time for a Normalization Process. Cat frying pans.*
>
> *Letter to My Friends + Family*
>
> *It's you fault you cunts ... Mother mostly it's your fault. You made me hate myself so much I cant stand my own mind. Thats why I'm filthy to keep you all away from the shit you made me experience myself as ... feeling my rage at your screwed up little mind ...*
>
> *If I'm clean you like me if you like me I feel good but ... there's a terrible terrible danger of love desire getting in I don't like that ... panic persecution. Take Vitamin B3 ... I'm taking off. I feel about as light as a balloon I'm taking off I can't write anymore I'm going onto the ceiling I got a pair of your knickers on Mama. What d'you think of that and I got a pair of Daddys pissed stained pants on. I got'em underneath my hat ... Seeing flashing lights? Peoples faces changing? Been seing a shrink for years without any change? Take Vitamin B3. I hate you ...*

I told Tony that he desperately wanted to be close to me but was afraid of either my "totally" rejecting him or my liking him "too much". He was still refusing to wash and be clean, and he tried to keep people at a distance; he was also challenging me to accept him as he was, with all his "shit". Wanting to be close to me produced in him feelings of panic and persecution. He wished he could just take something like Vitamin B3 and forget about everything; since he could not do that, he took off instead.

During this period in the treatment, Tony communicated with me mainly through these letters, sometimes very long ones, sometimes several in one session. He handed them over to me and closed his eyes. I usually read them straight away. On occasion I read only fragments of them or postponed reading them until later in the session. He still refused to speak. Perhaps this was not such an unwise decision, otherwise the delusional discourse that appeared in his letters would have been made explicit. He could not trust me enough yet. To write the words instead of speaking them created a transitional space that could be used by both of us. The emotional impact of the communication was mediated by the act of writing, by the paper, by the silenced words. Tony kept me safe from his delusional attacks while protecting himself from the possible re-enactment of an invasive mother who did not allow any privacy.

Tony's states of mind oscillated between psychotic and non-psychotic periods, but most of the time these two parts of himself seemed to coexist. Even during the intensely psychotic periods, he did not seem to deny reality. In the psychotic patient whose denial of reality is successful, one can assume that there is no room for phantasies or dreams; the psychic space is colonised by hallucinations. In fact, the appearance of dreams might be a sign of progress in the treatment, of reality becoming more acceptable. Nevertheless, Tony seemed to have phantasies and he also had dreams; he just did not report them.

This is another letter from that period:

> *I'm writing under the gaze of your fucking stupid all knowing cunt psychiatrist eye … You are the most beautiful woman I have ever met … We will go down to the sea. You+I … An exploding sunrise I will lick you cock and lie gazing as the sky. All the love in the world will pass between us. We will dissolve into the sky. Carnage+butchery*

> *I bear within my soul ... I want you to be my best friend no I don't ... Its like I'm hitting an iron door with a feather. I want to scream but I can't in your room ... I can't say how much I hate you you don't exist you mean nothing to me ... You are like glue your prick is made of glue I masturbate I really masturbate spunk flows into towels onto floors bits of lavatory paper sheets I covered my sheets in spunk it dried hard I used to wonder what my mother thought I'll send it to you for Christmas The world is dead ... I will tie you up and shit on you If you start saying "You want to do this because ... Youre telling me this because ..." then I will kill someone ... You must let me be your son Can this boy survive three days without his therapist?*

It was difficult for Tony to experience me as a stable, good object. I was not even experienced by him as having the stability of a bad, persecuting object. In his experience, I simply changed from one to the other without any continuity. I could easily move from being an all-knowing cunt [male] psychiatrist to the most beautiful woman, from his best friend to his most dangerous enemy, from a deaf therapist to a sticky prick or an idealised father. Nevertheless, he used the experience of writing these letters as an attempt at reparation and self-healing; it was a great relief when I had something to say about them, when he felt I had understood.

Lastly, I will quote a fragment of another of his letters:

> *You are my father. I am the demented child. You have brought me into the world last Christmas ... If I come here in the middle of the night Why do you care? Do you care? Who are you? Explain. I'm in the room now you're reading the letter ... Do you accept my foot? Accept my love before I die ... I don't know when I'm being persecuted by my mother. I'm splitting up. Heat on my neck. Marlene Dietrich on a bad trip. I know why I'm angry. I don't see you often enough. All this is berserk. I'm pretty berserk.*

By then, he no longer seemed to be lost in his psychosis. When he wrote, "You are my father", for example, he knew this was impossible; yet, at the same time, this was not the mere expression of a wish. It was more like a concrete and immediate demand that could not and should not be refused. It became essential for me to understand, for example, that I could not speak of his wish to be my son. It was much more relevant to let him know that he could not be my son because I did not want it. The direct introduction of my own desire in this way created a necessary third term, an active agency that could not be denied or ignored, shattering the mirage of an imaginary unity between Tony and an idealised mother-imago. For Tony, this was a source of incredible pain and frustration; little by little, he came to accept that this pain was far preferable to the delusional satisfaction of his wishes. The fact that he could stand the pain progressively became a source of strength.

The reference to the foot in the letter was not arbitrary. Sometimes he would take off his shoes to sit in a yoga position on the floor, or lie down on the couch. The stench would almost drive me from the room. For a long time, no interpretation or direct intervention on my part changed his attitude about washing himself. The foot, like other body parts, was something experienced as alien to himself, as a "real" part that did not connect to him. I interpreted this state of bodily de-fusion as having originated in the context of an early non-loving relationship with his mother, who had been unable to invest the body of her baby with loving feelings. I told him as much, adding that he could not imagine me, or anyone else for that matter, caring for him in a loving way.

Tony experienced his body in bits and pieces; as a way of dealing with this, he wished to merge with me in a total agglutinated and amorphous unity. In some sessions, Tony would be fixed on a part of his body: looking at his knee, for example, or his hand. The same might happen with a picture on the wall of my consulting-room. He would then find it difficult to move on to other things, because he lost the original connection with the context in which these things existed. The links that we normally take for granted were missing in his mind: a hand was a hand, separated from the rest of his body; thus, it had no meaning. He would ask: "What is a hand for?" This was not a rhetorical or philosophical question. Any part of his body could potentially turn into a persecuting object. By concentrating his attention on one element, Tony's perceptual Gestalt was lost. It may help to think of this in terms of the lack of a coherent narrative while first making a film: shots recorded do not follow the order in which they will be edited for the final version of the film; the different scenes appear at that point disjointed, lacking coherence; they must be connected during the process of editing. *Raccords* are what make syntactic continuity possible from frame to frame in a film sequence: they heal the gaps in the narrative, avoiding unwelcome *coupures* (confusing cuts). Tony appeared to perceive the world like a movie where the *raccords* were missing; this was reflected in the way his thought processes were constructed and expressed.

For a very long time, in the analysis, Tony was not able to look at me, nor at the things in my consulting-room. If he did look at me, he felt that the distance between him and me would completely disappear. He felt that he could, if he wished, penetrate me with his gaze and destroy me. He imagined that I might want to do the same to him. Perception did not respect the object's integrity; the boundaries between subject and objects and between objects themselves could not be kept. Confusion and angst contaminated all perceptual experiences. In fact, every object perceived, or any apparently arbitrary or minute aspect of the object, could become, for him, too special, all-important, all encompassing. His perception could transform a small event into an enormously far-reaching, meaningful moment. Tony kept his eyes closed and his mouth shut, but reality always managed to impinge on him. To allow reality to be perceived reminded him of the strangeness of things, of his own sense of dislocation and displacement. What could he do but keep himself paralysed and the world at a distance?

In the treatment, writing letters confirmed his way of denying the separation between us: he pulled me out of my own private environment and forced me into his. His negativism was at work: refusing to talk had been a rejection of the terms I had put forward for the analysis. I did not mind, even when I had found his long silences and his despair very difficult. But it soon became clear that the experience of writing letters had been essential for the continuation of the treatment. He had been literally terrified of saying what came into his mind. For him, it was no effort to free-associate in writing. Writing down his thoughts, frustrating as it was, offered him a certain sense of control. Talking to me, as much as looking at me, were sources of great terror, for he felt that the boundaries between us would disappear.

Tony, in moments of omnipotence, felt superior to others, pleased with himself for being "different"; in many ways, he expected my admiration for being "better" than his "normal" mother and sister. And yet, he had little reason to feel proud of himself. He knew he was psychotic, felt completely lost in life, and experienced as a dangerous threat his intense wishes to kill himself and others. It took him some time to admit it, but he also felt profoundly ashamed of his madness. Nevertheless, it was clear that Tony had enough courage to break away from his *self-institutionalisation* (Kohon, 1999), fighting for his destiny in diverse ways. For example, he refused electroshock treatment at the psychiatric hospital; he asked to be treated by psychotherapy; writing letters or bringing his dreams for analysis were active efforts on his part to gain control over his destiny. Later on, he would declare that his mother and sister could have their madness back; that he was not going to hell, that his mother could go by herself. He desperately wanted to turn what could have been a pathetic fate into a hopeful destiny.

There was a third period of Tony's therapy, based almost exclusively on the analysis of his dreams. The move from writing letters to telling me dreams represented an important step in the development of his therapy. To tell me his dreams took more courage than writing: it was an invitation to me to share more of his internal world. Tony became capable of separating from the external objects that subjugated him in reality. It helped him to establish a sense of separateness that, even though extremely precarious, made him feel alive. Literally, this meant that he was capable of having a mind of his own. I was amazed to see how he started to be capable of contemplating thinking as an independent, exclusive, playful activity. This was not achieved easily: as soon as he caught himself enjoying his thoughts, Tony feared that his mother would discover them and read them. Nevertheless, he felt more hopeful; he could dare to defy an angry, jealous, paranoid mother who, in his experience, had kept a tight control over his mind throughout his life. Now, he felt that he could have his thoughts without somebody else guessing them. The capacity to have thoughts and to be able to hide them was the first step towards true emotional independence. Tony discovered that he could have his own secrets, which meant that he could lie, like anyone else, as well as tell the truth. This activity gave him enormous pleasure: it was like seeing a child with a new toy. The fact that he could think of the pleasure present in the activity of thinking made a large contribution to his recovery.

One particular dream illustrated this movement:

> *He was travelling on a train with an old woman, a stranger, who kept complaining about everything: the seating arrangements, the food, the temperature of the carriage. He did not know why, but he felt*

embarrassed, as if he were responsible for her. Everyone was looking; he felt more and more uncomfortable. He wanted to push her out of the train but realised that it was none of his business. Finally, the woman descended at a station. It was near the Botanical Gardens at Kew, close to his mother's house. He then realised he was on his way to a session.

He was especially pleased that he had not pushed his mother out of the train in the dream. He had felt murderous towards her so many times in the past, it was a relief not to have to experience the persecuting guilt those feelings had always provoked in him. The reference to the Botanical Gardens was perhaps the most important signifier in the dream. In a recent session, Tony had made fun of Prince Charles and his alleged habit of talking to plants. So now Tony had felt that he was leaving his mother's "prince" behind with her, while he was travelling along, away from his mother, towards his analytic session.

As he began to feel less paranoid, he started to do some work; his first job through an agency was cleaning private houses. Given his own problems with cleanliness, this was a real laugh. We discovered that we could share the humour in these things. In fact, irony and laughter then became important elements of the therapeutic relationship. I believe that had this not happened, had we not been able to laugh together, then Tony's analysis would have proved impossible.

The saner Tony became, the crazier his mother and sister looked. The relationship between Tony and his sister had always been based on anger, competition, jealousy, and rivalry; now the difference was that Tony seemed able to defend himself more effectively. In one of the fights he reported, his sister started punching him, shouting, "You're psychotic! You're psychotic!" At this point, Tony was definitely not psychotic. He said in that session, "Now I know that my madness is their madness; they can have it back." His sister's frustration at not being able to win an argument by intimidating Tony, as previously, made her wish that "things could be like they used to be".

As I mentioned at the beginning, his mother had originally agreed to pay for Tony's therapy for one year, extended thereafter to a second. After that, Tony managed to pay for his own treatment. I agreed to keep my fees low until he was able to earn his living; this went on for several years, after which he paid my regular fee. Tony's mother seemed to find his growing independence very difficult: she tried to undermine his therapy and interfere in his relationship with me. For example, she would make ironic comments about his therapist or sarcastic remarks about the progress of the therapy. Tony felt caught up in the conflict; he thought his mother was trying to seduce him away from me; he felt guilty towards both his mother and me; his mother accused me of "taking her boy away", of turning her into a bad mother. At one point during the sixth year of therapy, she sent the following poem to him:

A SONG FOR MY SON
Let you concern yourselves with my son
For he is mad.
He stands apart and out of his eyes fall
Suns and stars. Galaxies
Pour through his veins, but blood is on his lips
His life bleeds from his lips.
His cries shriek out from The Abyss
He yearns to be again
Nothing and All,
The stuff of Creation before the first Sun
Frenzied Nothing with Fire …
You raise you dry eyes
Laugh at the riding boy of unreason
And your laugh is loud and terrible
More sad than your tears of the wandering, riding madman …
He r{e}aches my hands in headlong his high fight
Shrieking ecstasies "Come drink my blood of Light
Drink and be mad with ecstasies of fire
Of winds of water – lightning and the howling sea"
His blinding light unblinds my blindness
One moment. Oh almost I reach the flaming hands
Almost ride the airless furnace of the Void
with the Boy of madness and truth
Know flow through my fingers the sand of the stars
When my son's tears fall over unborn constellations …

The impact of this poem on Tony was staggering: it provoked one of the most regressive reactions of his analysis. It made him feel that, whatever progress he had made, he was not going to be able to change his relationship with his mother; something in him was going to stay mad forever.

Tony was made to believe and compelled to interpret the love of his mother as something exclusive. The baby might indeed want to be the exclusive object of maternal love, but to remain fixated to this omnipotent desire is the wish of the psychotic. Tony's mother tried to convince him that her love for him excluded everyone else: no father, no other child (sister) seemed to occupy such a privileged place in his mother's heart. The only object of the mother's desire was Tony. She was interfering and seductive, always demanding, always telling him what to do and how to be: his mother was never absent. He suffered all his life the terror of being taken over and overwhelmed by this powerful maternal object, his own personal "influencing machine" (Tausk, 1919). He was always too excited, anxious, on edge. By turning Tony into a baby desired and created by the royal family, the mother's discourse did not include her own desire, nor did she include a father with a desire of his own; there was no father whose desire would take mother away. Unable to cathect the sexual relationship with her husband, Tony's mother related to Tony through a process of idealisation of his origin, effectively depriving him of his true origin; she could not tell him, "You are my prince". Thus, a sense of belonging eluded Tony; it did not speak to him: he was alien to his life.

The question forced upon human beings by the Oedipus story is not only the triangular tragedy of rivalry, jealousy, and love, but also the drama of mis-recognition (*méconnaissance*) of their own history: Oedipus is the son of Jocasta and Laius, but he does not know it. In not being able to recognise his own history, he cannot identify or know his desire. Tony's fantasised origin did not refer to Tony himself; it spoke of his mother's own deluded origin. A father did exist, if only to have been killed in reality by Tony, according to his mother's version. But this man had nothing to do with either mother's desires or a desire of his own for the mother. The representation offered by the mother of the parents' sexual encounter was one not of mutual desire but of two desires, mother's and father's, rejecting each other.

Through his mother's poem Tony was thrown back once again into a confused state and could not discriminate which madness belonged to whom. He was convinced that he had driven his mother crazy. This terrified him: his own madness could drive me crazy. He wanted to stop the treatment; he claimed that it was all a waste of time and money. He became paranoid again and thought that people were following him around in underground stations; he felt ill and physically weak. He imagined raping his mother at his sister's place, of biting her tongue out while kissing her on the mouth. He became intensely jealous of anyone who approached or talked to his new girlfriend; he was convinced that because of his regression she was going to leave him. He could not bear the presence of any other patient in the waiting room; he was aggressive and nasty to other people when passing them on the stairs. He could not distinguish whether he was having all these bad feelings because of his own problems or because, he suggested, he was becoming his mother. He seriously thought of killing her. In one session, he reverted to writing letters:

> *I can't talk but I keep thinking things like your mother wouldn't like it if you didn't care for her I wouldn't like it if she didn't care for me I can't get it in my head it's terrifying I can't believe my mother hates me or I hate her. Remember I'm not a vicious man. I'm not bad. Yet he was hitting me he did hate me now you know what it felt like when your father saw you with your mother … They wouldn't admit they were wrong Somewhere they're such a lie fucking hell I'm in hell … My father is dead because I didn't help him in the garden. My mother said: "I remember a few days before he died working so hard in the garden – and you wouldn't help him". I killed my old man, anyone who kills their old man is a bastard … I just cut myself this is my blood* [there were, in fact, dried bloodstains on the paper] *I was thinking of suicide … That word SPLIT is dead right I'm writing to stay alive You inhuman charlatan I'm warning you This letter reminds me of the beginning when I first knew you … You can't even speak English. How the hell can it work when you can't even speak fucking English … I need to be able to hate her.*

At the beginning of his treatment, Tony had a strong wish to be dead – a wish described by Laing as the result of a primary guilt, originating in the feeling that one has no right to live. Tony "played dead" for a long time; he believed that if nothing moved, if he were able to keep things immobile and frozen, he could survive forever. If he were "dead", he could not die, nor could he kill (Laing, 1960). Indeed, at the start of the treatment I thought of Tony as being dead-in-life. The psychoanalytic task of giving meaning to the psychotic patient's utterances in the analytic encounter could be summarised thus: who would bring life to what, and for whom?

At times, I was afraid that Tony would actually kill himself, but I was reassured by the fact that he had never actually attempted suicide. I was more concerned that he would choose to withdraw completely, become truly catatonic. He felt a genuine terror of living. He wanted to anticipate danger and control his fears by entering a kind of psychic hibernation; he would then be able to hold on to his objects forever, never experiencing any loss. However, the term "experiencing a loss" would not describe Tony's feelings accurately; it was, rather, a fear of disintegration, a destruction of his being, a real catastrophe. To this he opposed the omnipotent fantasy of paralysing time, eliminating the differences between being alive and being dead. He lived in a permanent state of ontological contradiction. He experienced himself as living at both extremes of an emotional spectrum, encompassing impotence as well as omnipotence. While at a given moment he felt at the centre of the universe, determining and controlling the movements of people and the shape of things to come, he also imagined himself at the capricious mercy of malevolent external agencies. Every emotion, every affect, every fantasy was always matched by its opposite. Solipsistic grandeur was accompanied by the loss of a sense of self. Euphoria, secretly created by a well-guarded feeling of being in control of the universe, was matched by the nausea caused by the imaginary destruction of the world.

Nevertheless, patients seem to possess at times an inner organisation that helps them to modify original failures. I witnessed in Tony "the basic urge that patients have towards becoming normal" (Winnicott, 1965, p. 126). If transference is repetition, following thus the unconscious designs of the death instinct, it also creates the possibility for something new, something different, a new beginning.[4] In the context of the analytic encounter, a very special, unique intimacy develops between patient and analyst. Whatever happens in the transference situation is unpredictable, and the same can be said of love. Love is not just a repetition of a pattern from the past. An analysis might allow for new love objects to emerge, but, as Loewald (1960) has shown, it would be more relevant to think in terms of the analytic process facilitating a new discovery of objects, rather than a discovery of new objects.

The opportunity of analysing how he felt invaded and driven mad by his mother helped Tony to get through this period. He realised that his mother was insensitive to his needs, and this, far from being a mere product of his internal world, reflected the reality of the situation. The way in which he split the world into extremes of good and bad was an attempt to keep some sanity in the mother, some belief that she was not as horrible as she seemed. But he had to reconcile himself to the possibility that she might be as bad as he thought she was. He had believed in the past that his mother spoke a strange language: that he could not understand what she said. He was afraid that my own use of the English language was proof of my own insensitivity towards his needs. He also wanted to attack me with something that would really hurt me; he wished he could demean and belittle me.

The regressive episodes that Tony suffered were yet another reminder of how much he needed me. Tony was ashamed of his psychotic self. His dependence on me and his passionate transference-love for me humiliated him; he desperately wanted to make me feel the same way. The intensity of his feelings provoked in me a powerful sense of guilt: I felt I had let Tony down, betrayed him, that I should have been able to protect him from his mother.

In treating patients like Tony, the analyst cannot limit interpretations to the unconscious phantasy of the patient; what is also required is a specific acknowledgement of the reality of the actual dynamics of the therapeutic encounter. What I mean is that, in circumstances like these, it seemed necessary for me to recognise that I was in effect unable to protect Tony, and only then could I proceed with analytic interpretation. To give an example: it is the difference between saying to a patient, "Perhaps you feel that I cannot protect you from your mother", and saying, "The dilemma is that I cannot protect you from your mother, that I cannot be there with you, which is the only way you believe you would feel protected, that you could survive." Otherwise, I believe that a psychotic patient can hardly trust the analyst to understand him.

The subsequent period of the analysis was fruitful. Tony realised how much he needed to separate from the maternal body in which he had been trapped. As much as he wanted to live in a beatific, delusional unity with his mother, psychosis was too high a price to pay. "My father is dead because I didn't help him in the garden. My mother said ..." It was the word of the mother, establishing a false order of things: guilt, submission, emotional terrorism – but no real recognition in the mother of a word that belonged to the father. His father had lived in the shadows of his own past; according to Tony's mother, *that* first woman had never left his father's mind; whether this was true or not, the father's previous marriage had been the subject of innumerable arguments between him and Tony's mother. Consequently, it seemed that he had no place in the unyielding psychotic bubble that mother and son had formed; his father belonged to another family constellation, to the first wife. Tony had lived with the delusion that he could be everything for mother, but now he began to discover that this had been his mother's original wish. What had appeared to be an intense oedipal drama was a deceptive pantomime: Tony could not love his mother because she did not exist for him in any separate way. Nor did he exist for his mother. He could not own his own words: it was his mother who had said that he had killed his father. He did not know what place he occupied in a triangle: he was a royal prince, with no father; he had been given to mother for her own satisfaction. For Tony, to have the surname of his father did not identify him as his father's son; he felt outside the movement of the generations. He accepted these interpretations.

Access to his humour depended on Tony's moods, which were subject to great variation. Through his capacity for humour, Tony created a self-contained psychic environment where the madness of his mother could be kept at bay, excluded, in an area outside the self. If, at certain times, he would make fun of his mother's madness, humour served the essential purpose of enabling Tony to laugh at himself. There was also an implicit acknowledgement, present in both of us, that this was a precarious enterprise: there was no guarantee that the other would actually laugh at a given humorous intervention. Jokes and laughter could emerge at the most painful times, and I was wary of "celebrating" what could have been manic reactions on Tony's part. Humour was also part of a literary sensitivity that made Tony appreciate the writings of the Comte de Lautréamont, André Breton, Dylan Thomas, Rimbaud, Allen Ginsberg, and Charles Baudelaire, as well as punk rock, the Ramones, Luis Buñuel, and Latin American writers like José Donoso and Gabriel García Márquez. While punk rock and the Ramones' music and lyrics on madness never appealed to me, Tony's literary and cinematic preferences gave us a common ground where mutual processes of identification were possible.

In the middle of his process of recovery, Tony received yet another long letter from his mother. I will only quote a short fragment:

> *DANGER!! Jocasta calling!! If youve got 2 p to spare & an inclination to oblige an old geyser shed much appreciate – If not – forget it. Things arent at all up to mark here at Thebes. The latest trouble is that bloody sphinx. Blatantly neglecting her duties especially in her aspect of destructive Maternal Force. Shes been openly saying "Who does Zeus think he is anyway lobbering me with such a job in the first place & then underpaying me with all those jobs Ive had to devour because they were too thick to answer a damn silly riddle. They've given me serious stomach trouble* … [She ended the letter thus:] *Given at Thebes BC 1000 or there about a few centuries one way or another Jocasta Regina."*

Tony could not find any humour in this. Consequently, after a few sessions he felt profoundly sad about his mother and said to me: "She is mad, but I'm not going to sacrifice myself for her. If she wants to go to hell, let her, she's going alone. Let her burn, let it be fire." By then, he was having four sessions per week; it was at this point that the nature of the therapeutic work in Tony's analysis truly changed. Still, it took another few years for us to part. During that time he continued to move between a paranoid-schizoid and a depressive mode of being, but he was well aware of his own limits and how easily, for example, he could become anxious and paranoid. However, he was never psychotic again; he no longer experienced delusions, hallucinations, or "thought disorders".

Once Tony had found his way to my consulting-room, he proved to be psychologically minded. He offered me the opportunity to treat somebody who, while being seriously disturbed and for a long while psychotic, was able to respond to psychoanalytic treatment. Tony considered mental hospitals and the people working in them as part of a much-hated establishment, which included other figures of authority: the police, doctors, priests, the government, judges, and lawyers. This antagonism was one of the manifest reasons for refusing psychiatric treatment and seeking psychotherapy instead. He was helped by a mother, who, while very disturbed, was histrionic enough to wish to be seen by her children as "cool" and enlightened. After the death of his father, Tony had felt that his life had ended: he withdrew into himself, became a "loser" at school, could not see any future for himself; he was going to become a bum, a cripple, a dropout. Nevertheless, he was not yet psychotic. Only after taking drugs was he pushed over the edge towards a mental breakdown. At that point, he could possibly have ended up as a patient in a psychiatric institution. I have known several cases of people with a similar initial psychotic presentation who became, perhaps unnecessarily, more-or-less chronic psychiatric patients. Some of these cases were seriously disturbed, with a florid psychotic presentation at the beginning of the treatment; others suffered from consecutive acute episodes. I was lucky and grateful that Tony had accepted my offer of therapy. For his part, Tony was also grateful: he, too, considered himself to have been lucky and referred several times to the element of chance that had brought us together – chance enough to determine our fate, as Freud would have it (1910, p. 137).

At an early stage in his analysis, Tony quoted a Rolling Stones' song, reminding himself that one can't always get what one wants. Towards the end of his analysis, he thought he had got some of the things he needed to make life worth living. He developed further a small business he had started during the treatment, bought himself a house, had a girlfriend, and lived an independent life. Nevertheless, there was no happy ending; we both knew and acknowledged that these were not things that proved his sanity, nor were they the result of a complete cure. He was prone to serious periods of depression, but these did not prevent him from enjoying himself and his freedom. It was to Tony's credit that he was able to accept the irony of the psychoanalytic situation: he created me as the object that he needed, but then he had to reconcile himself to the fact that I was not it. He renounced the omnipotence of his wishes.

Love, in the time of madness, managed to keep "one up" on psychosis. When the analysis came to an end, we both knew that it could have gone on forever.

Notes

1 Rosenfeld (1987) mentioned this form in passing, but, as far as I know, he did not elaborate on it.

2 I think that this difficulty, to believe that the analyst *really* exists, may also be present on occasions in non-psychotic patients. For example, it may occur in-between one session and the next or during a weekend break. It can take the form of an uncanny feeling, believing and not believing, at one and the same time, that the analyst is a real person, creating a sense of depersonalisation in the subject.

3 The letters have been reproduced in their original spelling.

4 See my comments on the compulsion to repeat in Kohon (2019).

3

"BARBARA"

A symbiotic identification with an omnipotent mother imago

The night before she came to see me for her first consultation, "Barbara" had gone to bed with a stranger. She had been conscious throughout the evening that she would have to tell me about this the following day. In the morning she felt angry, abused, ill-treated: in her mind, she had become an enslaved sexual object in the man's tyrannical hands. She wished to disown responsibility for the event, as if the man had been guilty of getting her drunk, but she knew enough to admit to herself that she needed help. She felt frustrated: only a few days earlier she had thought that she did not need psychoanalysis; after all, if only briefly, she had the illusion of "getting her life together". Now, she had to face the harsh reality of promiscuity, of having lost her way in life. The feeble attempt at self-idealising denial ("I do not need analysis") soon crumbled into an accretion of confused feelings and chaotic actions that made Barbara acknowledge that she lived in a mess of her own creation. The pendulum movement between these contradictory self-perceptions (idealisation vs. denigration) was to be played out during the whole analysis. During the initial interview, her demand for treatment seemed genuine enough. "I was getting rid of you even before I started the analysis", she said. This could be considered the first interpretation in her treatment.

Barbara came from a small seaside town in Northern Australia, a place of great contrast between the world of white Australians and that of the "blacks" – as the Aboriginal people were referred to. Her parents were a typical lower-middle-class family. Proud and prejudiced, uneducated and bigoted, father was the "boss", mother was the "slave". They were dedicated church-goers, and much of their social life centred on the activities of their local church. Whenever he was not working in his hardware store, her father would spend his time watching TV, drinking at the pub, going fishing, or hunting with his mates. Her mother cleaned the house, cooked the meals, washed the clothes, went to church, and drank beer from morning until she dropped into bed at midnight. And yet, they were seen as pillars of the local community.

Barbara went travelling around the world after her mother's terminal illness was diagnosed. When her mother's condition worsened, she could have flown back to see her, but she was too indecisive: her mother died without Barbara being able to say goodbye. Although her mother was devalued by her father, Barbara remembered her as a powerful, omnipotent, simultaneously protective and persecuting presence in her life – a highly idealised figure with whom she had a very "unusual" relationship. She felt tortured by guilt towards her mother, persecuted by the idea that she had let her down, that she had not loved her enough. And, worse, had she wanted her dead?

After her mother died, her father did not wait long to marry a younger woman. This was a perfect match, according to Barbara: "She just does what he says, whatever he wants, she is his new slave." Her father hated blacks, but he also disliked independent women, feminists, and "lesbos"; above all, he could not stand "women who talked too much".

Barbara was depressed and felt lost. She had great difficulty in trusting anybody. Her sexual promiscuity and her tendency to erotise all relationships were effective ways of avoiding any real contact with others, leaving her feeling acutely empty. The thought of being in a close, intimate relationship threw her into a panic, making her feel unsafe and threatened. Instead of offering reassurance, pleasure, or fun, relationships were turned into battlegrounds where she fought imaginary wars. As much as she apparently desired it, human contact was toxic and dangerous. Grudges of one sort or another dominated her emotional life. The list of offences and transgressions that justified her rancour was comprehensive; her personal struggles were devoted to a search for magical solutions that never materialised. Always frantic and anxious, never leaving any proper mental space for herself, Barbara crowded her daily life with meetings, trips, events – an erotisation of chaos. During sessions she would talk compulsively or suddenly cry without consolation. She was chronically late, occasionally allowing herself only five or ten minutes of her session. She claimed that this left her feeling like a "slave" to her own neurosis.

The limits imposed by the psychoanalytic setting soon became a source of resentment. Despite having accepted the referral from the GP with relief and making considerable conscious efforts to commit herself to the treatment, she could not fully reconcile herself to her need for the analysis. "I don't want to become enslaved to this process", she claimed. Nevertheless, her rebellion against the analytic process and her defensive behaviour took place in the context of a hidden and yet most compelling transference. For a long time, she could not talk about it, but ultimately she declared that she was "in love" with me; desperately, and yet feeling hopeless, she also wanted me to love her. Towards the end of the third year of treatment, she was "delayed" gathering her things from the waiting room, and she met my next patient, a young man arriving on a bicycle. Surprisingly, she came to the following session on time. She reported having been extremely distressed by meeting the other patient; she was tormented by jealousy, she said, and was afraid of going mad. Then she withdrew into silence for the rest of the session.

At the next session, she brought the following dream:

> *She was falling into a black hole; she was scared to death; she felt that nobody could help her, that nobody loved her enough to care. She went to her parents' bedroom; mother was there at first but then she disappeared. Instead, her brother was standing by the parents' bed, smiling. Then, he also disappeared. "Where had they gone?" she asked herself, "Was her mother dead?" No, her mother reappeared, naked, behind a net curtain by the window. She was taken aback by discovering that she woke up feeling sexually excited.*

In a rather arrogant way, adopting an incongruously posh accent, Barbara claimed to have been traumatised by the encounter with my other patient. Her brother's birth (when she was three years old) had been the one and only real tragedy in her life. "I hated him", she told me while sobbing furiously. At the time of her brother's birth, she was sent away for a few weeks to stay with a maternal aunt (her mother's twin sister) in a nearby town. The wretchedness she experienced was not compensated by the small presents she was given every night by her aunt and uncle, benign figures whose generosity, paradoxically, only added further to her misery. There was no solace or relief for the suffering little girl, just an intense distress: "I was the princess, the apple of my mother's eye. I never wanted to give that up, it was my place in the world, and my brother came to ruin it all."

Among other things, the dream vividly portrayed Barbara's pathological distortions of the primal scene. Confronted by the reality of parents having intercourse and making babies, Barbara appeared through her associations to conceive of the parental couple constituted by mother and brother, rather than mother and father. In Barbara's mind, while father was not given true existence, her brother was represented in the dream as a grown-up man, enjoying himself. She knew that the baby had been the product of sexual intercourse between her parents; after all, she was not psychotic. Nevertheless, she was utterly convinced that her relationship with mother had been, up to then, a "marriage made in heaven". At one and the same time, she seemed to affirm and deny that the brother had and had not arrived in this world as a consequence of her parents' intercourse. To the patient's own uneasiness and consternation, she woke up feeling sexually aroused after this dream of a primal scene in disguise, imagined as the sexual encounter of mother and brother.

A multiplicity of specific triangular scenes unfold in the telling of Barbara's story. They illustrate the complex and confused misrepresentations of the primal scene, envisaged exclusively as the arena for sadomasochistic scenarios, with different characters exchanging positions and playing alternative roles. We may imagine a theatrical sequence. In *Scene 1* we hear of the appearance of a stranger in the position of the abuser, Barbara becoming a slave to his tyrannical wishes. The third party is represented by the presence of the analyst in Barbara's mind, a reminder of her need for the analysis. In *Scene 2* we have another abuser, this time the father, forever ill-treating the mother, his slave. Barbara occupies the third place, a helpless witness to the parents' relationship. In *Scene 3* Barbara occupies the place of the abuser: this time she is the young traveller who leaves the mother (the suffering, ill slave) to die without saying goodbye to her. The third position seems to be occupied by Barbara's superego, accusing her of neglect. *Scene 4* brings father back to the position of boss, marrying another woman – his new slave – soon after the death of Barbara's mother. Barbara is the third party, witness and judge of her father's misdemeanour. After the list of "wrongs" that have been inflicted upon her, *Scene 5* places the story closer to home: this time the analyst seems to be the abuser; Barbara is the patient enslaved by the very analytic process; her GP is in the background, occupying the position of witness and judge. *Scene 6* shows Barbara reacting with a tantrum to meeting another patient in the waiting room. She becomes the slave abused by the analyst's assumed cruelty, accusing him of not protecting her enough. The other patient/analytic sibling/brother seems to be the witness to her fury. Finally, we arrive at the dream (*Scene 7*), where a couple in the bedroom make Barbara go through seemingly unbearable jealousy. In this last scene, at one point her mother and her brother disappear – perhaps an indication of murderous feelings previously repressed. Then, there is the sexual excitement when her naked mother reappears, while her brother remains absent, a focal point in Barbara's analysis. There is a *Scene 8*, central to Barbara's predicament, which I will leave for discussion later.

Barbara was powerfully invested in a primary identification with a maternal imago, which was experienced only in extreme terms: either as an idealised good object or as a thoroughly persecuting and/or damaged bad one. This constituted the psychic background, the main emotional and sexual scenario in which her object relationships were played out.

At times Barbara expressed the conscious wish that, "if only she was a man", she would not experience the lack of a penis, which she saw as the lack of the "only" anchoring point that would offer her a secure sense of identity. She feared that separating from mother would cause her mother to have a breakdown. Feeling that her body "belonged" to her mother, she suffered intense and frequent paranoid psychosomatic anxieties; paradoxically, this made her feel "united" to her mother, whom she would never have to leave … even if, in reality, she had managed to move almost 17,000 km away from her. In her imagination, Barbara conceived of her mother as someone who could and would want to damage her: fearing her mother's power to hurt her, to poison her, or to destroy her internal organs, including her genitals, made her feel extremely vulnerable. Simultaneously, her mother's aggressive impulses, imaginary or real, and the dreaded primary phantasies of being incorporated, eaten, and swallowed and disappearing back into the mother resulted in the tendency to suppress her own aggression, to submit and conform too much – this becoming an important factor in the development of her masochism (Halberstadt-Freud, 1989).

Laplanche and Pontalis refer to the "rare occasions" (1967, p. 336) when Freud used the concept of primary identification. Although in *Group Psychology and the Analysis of the Ego* (1921) Freud had spoken of a primitive type of identification where the difference between self and object had not yet taken place, there seems to be only one instance in the *Standard Edition* when he specifically used the expression "primary identification". In *The Ego and the Id*, Freud wrote that "the effects of the first identifications made in earliest childhood will be general and lasting" (1923, p. 31). We could understand this as a simple reference to identification with the primary objects. Many authors have understood it as such and rejected this notion. Their main objection can be summarised thus: that it would not make sense to invoke a concept of "identification" when there is not yet an emotional tie to a differentiated object with whom to identify (Blum, 1973).

From a different point of view, de Mijolla defended the Freudian concept of primary identification – one that, most significantly, he called ontological. Acknowledging how difficult it is sometimes to define or determine them, he spoke of "unconscious identification fantasies", describing them as

> imaginary constructions or even veritable unconscious fantasmatic scenarios by means of which a subject substitutes a primordial character from his family history, especially father, mother or grandparent, for a part of his ego or superego.
>
> (Mijolla, 1987, p. 399)

De Mijolla suggests that this identification takes place during pregnancy, where both parents are reviving stories of their individual past. The impossibility of representing the growing foetus inside the womb creates a psychic vacuum that is filled with unconscious emotions and phantasies projected onto the yet-to-be-born baby. The return of the repressed from the past of the parents and grandparents (as well as of other members of the family) will mark the baby's own psyche. It is never just money, clothes, precious jewellery, or significant first names that children inherit from previous generations. At the infant's birth, for example, various members of the different families might claim, "this baby is the spitting image of ...", demonstrating their own emotional investment in the new creature, their speculative meanders forming the basis of a fantasmatic projection onto the newborn. More crucially, and perhaps more critically, these projections might include unconscious phantasies concerning previous deaths in the family, mourning processes that have not been worked through, identifying designations (de Mijolla argues) that "can later reinforce the rigid mould in which a nascent ego can become petrified if the psychic violence exceeds the defensive possibilities each subject possesses ..." (1987, p. 400).

Freud had something different in mind. For him,

> This [primary identification] is apparently not in the first instance the consequence of the outcome of an object-cathexis; it is a direct and immediate identification and takes place earlier than any object-cathexis.
>
> (Freud, 1923, p. 31)

Freud argued for the consideration of "an organization which was a slave to the pleasure principle and neglected the reality of the external world ...". Our logic tells us that this organization, as he said, "could not have come into existence at all" (Freud, 1911, p. 219). And yet, he added,

> The employment of a fiction like this is, however, justified when one considers that the infant – provided one includes with it the care it receives from its mother – does almost realize a psychical system of this kind. It probably hallucinates the fulfilment of its internal needs; it betrays its unpleasure, when there is an increase of stimulus and an absence of satisfaction, by the motor discharge of screaming and beating about with its arms and legs, and it then experiences the satisfaction it has hallucinated. Later, as an older child, it learns to employ these manifestations of discharge intentionally as methods of expressing its feelings.
>
> (Freud, 1911, p. 219)

Could we conceive of such an auto-erotic psychic organisation, characterised by drives and affects that will not easily or necessarily ever be the object of conscious representation? Perelberg, among other authors, has referred to the unconscious imago of a phallic all-powerful mother that is, she argued, present in the early psychic life of both girls and boys (Perelberg, 1997, pp. 21–23).[1]

A girl has contradictory desires: on the one hand, for the development of a separate identity and a sexuality of her own and, on the other, an intense, extreme wish for a special unity with her mother. Halberstadt-Freud (1989) coined the term *symbiotic illusion* to describe the potential existence of a primary identification between mother and daughter from the very beginning of life, before the development of object relations; this identification would interfere with, or even prevent the formation of a separate identity for the girl. Later in life, a woman's development and the struggle to separate from mother become problematic: every step towards independence is accompanied by conflict, leading to a propensity to regress to earlier phases. Separation becomes a source of guilt, shame, a sense of disloyalty, and may become an act of aggression against the mother.

Object relationships are there from the beginning of life outside the womb. But would this truly eliminate any consideration of a retroactive re-edition of a monadic structure closed in upon itself, prior to the separation of self and other, preceding any possibility of a sexual division, and characterised by a sense of completion—an illusory form of self-sufficiency, as described by the concept of primary narcissism?

The concept of primary narcissism denotes, according to Laplanche and Pontalis, "an early state in which the child cathects its own self with the whole of its libido" (1967, p. 337). As they acknowledged, this is a rather unsatisfactory definition. There are many different and contrasting definitions of the concept in the psychoanalytic literature. The theoretical and clinical obstacles are multiple: how can we agree upon the existence of this hypothetical stage of development? What would be its chronological place? The mother's womb? If so, then what is being cathected? If it were an objectless state, then how can we call it "narcissism", since, by definition, this term implies an image of the self?

The concept was rejected by most object relations psychoanalysts – except Winnicott. From Melanie Klein and Michael Balint onwards, most British analysts argued that the baby relates to objects from the beginning. Since the recognition of an external object is there from the very beginning of life, they claimed that the baby could not take his own ego as the first object. For them, the first object is the breast: therefore, narcissism would always be secondary – that is, a product of the internalisation of the idealised primary object.

Nevertheless, primary narcissism designates a mythical state of primal plenitude. At this point, the baby is thought to have the illusion of complete omnipotence; its belief in the omnipotence of its thoughts is independent of the relationship to the primary object. It is conceivable that, while taking its own ego, or body, or self as its own ideal, the baby can still relate to an object from the beginning of life. This paradoxical state, where there is neither room for desire nor any sense of loss, is only interrupted and eventually fractured by the inevitable separation from the mother.

Bion spoke of "preconceptions": an innate disposition in the baby's mind to discover and find an object – for example, a pre-existing expectation that the mouth will find a nipple. This is not dissimilar to what Winnicott described as the "initial experience of omnipotence":

> We have to say that the baby created the breast, but could not have done so had not the mother come along with the breast just at that moment. The communication to the baby is: "Come at the world creatively, create the world; it is only what you create that has meaning for you". Next comes: "the world is in your control."
>
> (Winnicott, 1968, p. 101)

From a structural perspective, and once we relate them to Freud's concept of primary narcissism, Winnicott's own concepts of transitional objects and transitional phenomena can be more fully understood. He described the baby's ability to create the breast thus:

> … the breast is created by the infant over and over again out of the capacity to love or (one can say) out of need. A subjective phenomenon develops in the baby, which we call the mother's breast.
>
> (1951, pp. 238–239)

The existence of the object (breast, mother) in the external world does not exclude the experience of primary narcissism in the baby. Evoking similar attributes, Winnicott describes it as the stage of absolute dependence, both in terms of the baby's needing a womb in which to develop and in terms of the total care he requires once he is born. "In this state", Winnicott says, "the infant has no means of knowing about ... the maternal care ..." (1960b, p. 46). He has to "invent" it all through his omnipotence. Previously, Winnicott had defined it as "innate primary creativity" (1947a, p. 90).

The concept of primary identification would account for this pre-object state in which, following Lebovici's famous statement, "The object is cathected before being perceived" (1961, p. 151). If this were so, the hallucinated satisfaction of a need "must therefore be differentiated from hallucinating the object" (Gibeault, 2010, p. 272).

The theoretical and clinical consequences of this are significant. The existence of a primary identification in a pre-object stage would not exclude the crucial importance of the subject's object relationships. It is not a question of either/or. The condition for the survival (or re-edition) of this primitive identification will depend entirely on the vicissitudes of the primary object relationships. For example, a narcissistic over-investment in their baby by one or both parental figures will contribute to the subject's not being able to work through his/her own narcissistic identification. An intense and extended pathological narcissism in the mother would fail to provide the function of a protective shield (Khan, 1963), necessary to work through the prolonged initial stage of helplessness (Freud, 1926a). Instead, parents may create the delusional conviction in the baby that he does not need anybody; later on in life, the subject might be manically driven to deny the original sense of helplessness; it would appear as if there were only an idealised, good, all-giving breast: no disappointments here, only gratification. The inside world of the womb is extended to the notion of an omnipotent mother, a combined object that comprises the baby's internal world plus "[the mother's] voice, her face, her hands, and her bosom" (Kristeva, 2000, p. 63), which constitute the mother's bodily "presence" (Klein, Heimann, Isaacs & Riviere, 1952, p. 119).

If we now return to the concept of the maternal imago, we know that Freud used the word "imago" sparingly. In the writings of Melanie Klein, by contrast, it gained a special place at times – for example, when she described the "imagoes of the combined parents" present at the source of the most extreme anxieties. The importance that she gave to the concept became a significant part of her clinical descriptions. In her view, part of the work of the analysis consisted in turning the terrifying parental imagoes into more benign ones. It was left to Susan Isaacs to attempt to clarify the concept as an unconscious image of a person or part of a person, the earliest objects:

> In psycho-analytic thought, we have heard more of "*imago*" than of *image*. The distinctions between an "*imago*" and "*image*" might be summarized as: (a) "*imago*" refers to an *unconscious* image; (b) "*imago*" usually refers to a person or part of a person, the earliest objects, whilst "*image*" may be of any object or situation, human or otherwise; and (c) "*imago*" includes all the somatic and emotional elements in the subject's relation to the imaged person, the bodily links in unconscious phantasy with the id, the phantasy of incorporation which underlies the process of introjection; whereas in the "image" the somatic and much of the emotional elements are largely repressed.
>
> (Isaacs, 1948, p. 93)

Most significantly, in the context of the present argument, Isaacs' understanding of the concept of *imago*

> includes all the somatic and emotional elements in the subject's relation to the imaged person, the bodily links in unconscious phantasy with the id, [and] the phantasy of incorporation which underlies the process of introjection … .
>
> (Isaacs, 1948, p. 93)

Laplanche and Pontalis defined imago as an "Unconscious prototypical figure which orientates the subject's way of apprehending others …" (1967, p. 211). The complexity of the concept was further addressed by the authors thus: "It should be looked upon … as a stereotype through which, as it were, the subject views the other person" (p. 211).

I now return to Barbara's story. The associations to her dream revealed the impact of the birth of her brother, which was re-experienced in the situation of transference through the chance encounter with another patient. And yet the birth of her brother *per se* proved not to be the original trauma. There was the unsettling association between the birth of a sibling and her own "murder" and "death": while one child (brother) was born, another child (Barbara) was being killed. This was accompanied by another relevant admission: Barbara had a "secret" that, she claimed, she did not want to share with anybody; in fact, she had never mentioned it to anyone else. The idea occupied a shadowy and obscure pre-conscious place in her mind – it lived in a twilight zone. It was as if this was the first time this thought had become truly conscious to her, an eye-opener.

She confessed that "deep down" she believed herself to be a beautiful woman whom nobody could ever resist. One of her omnipotent wishes was that, in spite of her seemingly negative behaviour in the analysis, one day her analyst was going to realise what a wonderful baby she had been in the past and what an attractive woman she was in the present. She seemed utterly convinced that she had been – and was still – this marvellous child, with astonishing appeal and unusual intelligence. In her mind, Barbara and her mother lived together in "heavenly unity", an apparently idyllic time in a space of wonder and magic – that is, until her brother was born. Why did I not protect her from meeting my other patients? That was not fair, she said: everything could have been so "different" for us, patient and analyst. She expressed her wish for this "blissful union" to be re-created in the analysis with me. If she could not have that union with me, then there was no point: the analysis would not be of any use. She insisted on her intense love for me; "I could be your slave", she proclaimed, as much with anguish as with irony and excitement. "And nobody would know", she added.

We have here, finally, the missing *Scene 8*. In her unhappy life, Barbara wanted to recreate once again the perverse scenario of abuser/abused, suggesting she become the slave of the analyst, as if it were the only possible solution to her predicament. In this newly wished-for scenario, the third party was being represented by an absence: "nobody".

Barbara was under the ascendancy of a compulsion to repeat the structure of the original trauma: that of a symbiotic narcissistic relationship with an omnipotent mother imago, only imagined and reconstructed retroactively, expressed and verbalised by the patient after the experience of the dream. Confusing love and hate, birth and death/murder, wishing to ignore what she unconsciously already knew, she desired to be a slave once again. This compulsion made itself present in the transference through her desire to become the love-slave of her mother/analyst. The desire was not just to compensate for learning that there were other patients/siblings. Under normal circumstances, Barbara could have been, just as many others, "traumatised" by the birth of her sibling. The consideration of the birth of her brother as the most important traumatic event in her life helped her to "normalise" her distress. Nevertheless, this way of understanding her existential project left out the particular relationship she had been caught up in with her mother.

Barbara's mother had always claimed that sending Barbara to be with her own sister was a "great thing" because mother and sister were "the same": in her mother's mind, since they were twins, there was no difference between them. Before sending her away, during those first three years, Barbara could recall her mother addressing her as "my doll", while dressing Barbara both in girls' as well as in boys' clothes. No difference between the siblings, mother and her twin sister, nor between Barbara and her own brother; no real difference between the generations, and no sexual difference to speak of. All Barbara wanted was to restore and re-live the original narcissistic bubble, the idealised, symbiotic, quasi-delusional relationship with her mother. She wished to be the chosen princess/slave/patient – the only one – surrendering herself to the designs of her analyst in the context of a sadomasochistic relationship.

The magnitude of a primary trauma was recreated and could only be understood *après coup*: the extreme distress evoked by the encounter with another patient in the present gave authentic meaning to the sorrow of the past. And yet, it was this original unhappiness and despair that continued to determine Barbara's life in the present. The idealised "bubble" proved in reality to be a cyst full of poisonous secretions.

In one of her sessions, as she had done at other times, Barbara spent a considerable time complaining, criticising, and attacking her mother. Barbara spoke with strong conviction about a mother who was always unhappy, resentful, sadistically triumphant in the control of her daughter, and bitterly disappointed by her husband, by men, by humanity. It was not difficult to identify the same feelings of unhappiness in Barbara: the resentment towards her mother contaminated Barbara's relationships with the rest of her world. At that point, my interpretation addressed the question of how much the terrorism of the mother's depression exerted an uncanny fascination over Barbara; she remained entrapped in the meaningless world of her mother's psychic void. Barbara became noticeably tense on the couch. Turning around to face me, she furiously shouted, "*I* can say whatever I like about my mother but you cannot; *you* have no right to make such a … character assassination!"

This expression normally implies that the truth of the allegations and attacks made on a person is irrelevant. Had Barbara understood my interpretation as something too "concrete", as if I were referring a bit too much to the "reality" of the mother? For a brief moment, I felt rather depersonalised. At that moment, who had I become for her?

As I was recovering from her reaction, another thought came to mind– a thought that I did not put into words: "Is this what you have been attempting to do in the analysis, a (character) assassination of your mother?" *Attempting to* – and yet not being able to achieve it. *Assassination* – maybe, but no conception of a meaningful separation from her mother. Although Barbara desperately needed to leave her mother, she could not gain any significant distance from her. Furthermore, she could not imagine, in any fruitful or creative way, how to grow up and become a subject in her own right, capable of owning her own words. For Barbara, to relinquish the primitive involvement with mother was too concretely associated with the threat of actually murdering her.

In the end, although the dead body of her mother was kept in the hospital mortuary for a couple of weeks before finally being buried, Barbara did not dare to attend the funeral. There was a palpable and sinister sense of unconscious pleasure in Barbara's phantasising about her mother's dead body, imagining and visualising it on a stretcher in an empty room, her face still exposed, confusingly alive in death. The murdered mother had been introjected as a murderous internal object, locked up within herself, in a reversal that made Barbara forever melancholically miserable.

As Freud said of childhood memories, Barbara's memory was formed in the process of the analysis (1899, p. 322). The content of the story was created by the telling of it. The re-living of the trauma was a construction of the analysis and was only then turned into meaningful historical truth by the interpretative work of patient and analyst in the process of analysing the patient. Such an analytic construction does not necessarily mean that events surrounding a trauma did happen in the reality of the past. One could argue that, without the analysis, this trauma would have not existed in Barbara's telling of her story. Her history was mobilised, in Haydée Faimberg's words, by the very enigmas "posed by the transference" (2005, p. 7).

We could tentatively argue that primary unconscious identifications could be considered an essential factor in the constitution of the subject, a process that is structural rather than based only on object relationships. These identifications are not reducible to rational explanations or to common-sense descriptions; they are only discovered *après-coup*. Most importantly, there seems to be a primary projection of phantasies and unconscious feelings onto the very early parental figures. In other words, the very perception of the original primary figures may be distorted by unconscious phenomena. Different psychoanalytic authors have suggested a variety of concepts to describe this: imago (e.g., Klein, 1926, 1927, 1931, 1932, 1935, 1945; Lacan, 1953); schema (Piaget, 1973); archaic meaning schemata (Székely, 1962); primal phantasies (Freud, 1915b, 1916–17); pre-conceptions (Bion, 1962a, 1962b, 1963, 1965, 1970); primary matrices of phantasies (Chasseguet-Smirgel, 1995); fantasising function (Freud, 1924); primitive organising activity (Joffe & Sandler, 1979); primary unconscious narcissistic representations (Leclaire, 1975); radical imaginary (Castoriadis, 1987), and unconscious patterns.[2]

This perceptual distortion is an imaginary consequence that does not seem to have been created exclusively from actual personal experiences; nevertheless, it organises all early experiences and creates the possibility for meaning. Primary projections of phantasies may be symbolically unrecognisable in any direct form and only revealed by the unconscious through symptoms, dreams, and slips of the tongue and, more specifically, in the analytic setting through transference and acting-out. They do not exist without the establishment and development of a psychoanalytic dialogue. Since they cannot be translated into images, the hypothesis about their existence may be considered fanciful or even mythical, but it imposes itself on us as something theoretically indispensable (Bergeret, 1974).

In conclusion, on the one hand, in many female patients the presence of a primary identification with a maternal imago epitomises an all-powerful, sublime, awe-inspiring, protective, and sacred figure, a benign presence that could justifiably be described as "maternal". And yet, on the other hand, the same imago can personify a vulnerable, pathetic figure, dominated by helplessness, sadness, illnesses, and inhibitions that – perhaps as part of this negative side – can, nevertheless, be domineering, tyrannical, rancorous, and implacable. These contradictory extremes lie at the core of the subject's own narcissistic identifications. This mother imago is invested with an ideal of narcissistic omnipotence, seducing the subject into believing that there is a Paradise that not only should never have been lost but that constitutes the very self of the subject. The imago conveys the unconscious presence of a ubiquitous, internal, threatening breast, which may make the subject feel ostracised, inadequate, lacking, and displaced.

The unconscious reminiscence of the subject's connection and struggles with this primary imago constitute the mythical background against which the subject's object relationships will develop. Depending on the vicissitudes of the individual's personal history, this omnipotent and persecuting imago might be re-evoked, re-visited, and re-experienced subsequently in the subject's libidinal life. Following on from Freud's idea of trauma in the "Project" (1950 [1895]), this is only re-created, developed, and understood *après coup* through the work of analysis.

Notes

1 A list of authors, however incomplete, who have referred to this kind of mother imago includes, among others: Benjamin (1988); Bernstein (1983); Chasseguet-Smirgel (1964); Chodorow (1978); Deutsch (1932, 1944); Fast (1984); Fliegel (1973, 1986); Freud (1920b, 1931); Friday (1977); Galenson (1986); Galenson and Roiphe (1976); Halberstadt-Freud (1989); Horney (1924, 1926, 1932, 1933); Jones (1927, 1933, 1935); Klein (1926, 1928, 1932); Lampl-de Groot (1927); McDougall (1964, 1986); Roiphe and Galenson (1981); Stoller (1976); and Torok (1964).

2 According to PEP-Web, there are 10,000 possible references, in different variations, in the *International Journal of Psychoanalysis*.

4

BETWEEN THE FEAR OF MADNESS AND THE NEED TO BE MAD

Psychoanalysts tend to present to the public their successful cases, rather than their failures. Nevertheless, we still know relatively little about what really makes an analysis a success. Ironically, in spite of the abundance of psychoanalytic writings, it is easier to reflect on what makes it a failure.

I would like to reflect further on Tony and Barbara, whose case studies were presented in Chapters 2 and 3.

Joan Riviere tells us that one day during her analysis Freud made an interpretation to which she responded with an objection: "He then said: 'It is unconscious.' I was overwhelmed then", she confessed, "by the realization that I knew nothing about it" (Riviere, 1958). Any true psychoanalytic insight carries with it this feeling of being overwhelmed, not so much by the discovery of something new as by the fact that we did not know about it. Far from being a mere intellectual exercise or, conversely, a purely cathartic one, psychoanalysis demands from the patient, in the first place, a certain capacity for humility, which enables the subject to bear knowing so little about himself. This is independent of the presenting complaints, the degree of pathological disturbance, or the social circumstances. In the second place, psychoanalysis demands the existence of a *conflict of suffering* – not only "conflict" and not just "suffering". As far as I know, Freud only used the concept of *Leidenskonflikt* once, in a letter to Edoardo Weiss: he believed that only a conflict that provoked suffering can motivate the subject to look for a cure. Then Freud proceeded to make the unusual suggestion that one should get rid of those patients who do not suffer. One should "ship them overseas, let us say to South America, and let them look for and find their destiny there" (Freud & Weiss, 1920, p. 49).

Tony, although highly disturbed, proved that he could fulfil these two requirements: he was capable of humility, and he felt enough motivation through his suffering to search for and accept therapeutic help. While Barbara had searched for help through her suffering, she found it much more difficult to relent, to give up a psychic organisation that was experienced by her as protecting her self-identity. It could be argued that these two patients shared a similar, if still different, psychic disposition. They both experienced, in different ways, intense terrors that were based on phantasies of being invaded, annihilated, losing their selves "into" others.

There is yet a third important condition required by psychoanalysis that Tony fulfilled: what Freud described as the possession of a "fairly reliable character" (1905, p. 263). As Guy Thompson has remarked, "the need for a reliable character can't be emphasised too highly". He rightly argues that this is a "prerequisite of treatment, not its consequence" (Thompson, 1994, p. 156). In other words, a poor character cannot be treated: chronic liars and pathological deceivers, for example, cannot overcome their lies and their deceptions. Nina Coltart was one clinician who gave explicit importance to moral character and/or ethical reliability in the clinical assessment of patients for psychoanalysis (Coltart, 1987). Once, when referring to me a patient who, I argued, was too disturbed for analysis, Coltart insisted: "Maybe, but he is *decent*."

In *The Question of Lay Analysis* (1926b), Freud described fairly common human situations as part of the motivation to seek psychoanalytic treatment: fluctuations in moods, a sense of despondency and insecurity, "nervous embarrassment among strangers", "difficulties in carrying out his professional work", "feelings of anxiety", inhibition from walking on the streets alone or travelling by train, headaches, fainting spells, difficulties with their sexuality. People went to doctors, who offered them ineffectual forms of treatment that gave them temporary relief, or none at all. When eventually the disappointed patients arrived at the analyst's consulting-room, they were faced with the fact that, "Nothing takes place between [patient and analyst] except that they talk to each other" (1926b, p. 187).

A patient, Freud continued, had to accept the existence of "things in himself that he would be very unwilling to tell other people ... and other things that one would not care to admit to oneself". This already represented a "great advance in psychological self-knowledge", but then something else happens: "a very remarkable psychological problem begins to appear". In the situation of treatment, the patient becomes aware

> of a thought of his own being kept secret from his own self. It looks as though his own self were no longer the unity which he had always considered it to be, as though there were something else as well in him that could confront that self.
>
> (Freud, 1926b, p. 188)

It is this notion, that there is no unity within one's self, that constitutes for some the most revolutionary aspect of Freud's ideas (Rorty, 1989, 1991). When the subjects in analysis are capable of accepting the existence of a psychic reality alien to themselves, when they recognise that their self contains something secret or different or contradictory to their wishes and thoughts and that this something might be part of a conflict that is making them suffer, we say that they are psychologically minded (Coltart, 1987, 1988). The patients can then contemplate the idea that anything that takes place in that psychic scenario, even the most inexplicable psychological event, might have meaning and thus is worth thinking about. Absurd dreams, the strangest of symptoms, contradictory memories that seem to come from nowhere, or bizarre thoughts arising from events of everyday life, they are all the result of a dynamic process that originates in an area of darkness, the consequence of unconscious conflicts unknown to us. The analyst is not there to teach the meaning of her actions to the patient; the analyst is not there to "cure" the patient, indoctrinate, or save him. Instead, through listening, the analyst tries not to interfere with the mutual process of learning from the other. The patient's speech becomes meaningful through the analyst's listening, which changes the narrative offered by the patient. It is never the same to tell a dream to a friend or a spouse as to tell it to one's analyst, but it is not the analyst who creates the meaning of the dream for the patient. The unconscious meaning unfolds exclusively through the discourse of the patient, revealed, as it were, by the analyst's capacity to listen.

When Tony started therapy with me, I was involved with what was known as the anti-psychiatry movement in the United

Kingdom, and I had lived for a time with psychotic people in a small therapeutic community in Archway, North London. My previous training in the late 1960s as a clinical psychologist in Argentina had been profoundly influenced by psychoanalysis. Although at that time non-medical people were not allowed to train at the then only Argentinean psychoanalytic institute, psychologists were taught at the university and were privately encouraged, supervised, and analysed by members of the local psychoanalytic society, who were, then, mainly Kleinian. Through the influence of the writings of Wilfred R. Bion, Hanna Segal, and Herbert Rosenfeld, the visits of British analysts, and the teachings of people like Enrique Pichon-Rivière and José Bleger, it was not unusual for clinicians to treat disturbed patients in their private psychoanalytic practices. Pichon-Rivière had published his paper on "Psicoanálisis de la Esquizofrenia" in 1947, the same year that Rosenfeld published his first paper on the "Analysis of a Schizophrenic State with Depersonalization" (1947). This was only one year after Melanie Klein's "Notes on Some Schizoid Mechanisms" (1946). Pichon-Rivière had also been one of the official presenters at the XIV Congrès des Psychoanalystes de Langue Française, where he read his paper "Quelques Observations sur le Transfert chez des Patients Psychotiques" (1952). In similar fashion to his Kleinian colleagues from Europe, Pichon-Rivière thought that, in spite of their extreme defensive withdrawal from reality, schizophrenic patients were capable of intense transferences. He believed that their treatment should be centred on the analysis of the transference and the mechanism of projective identification.

At the beginning of my practice in London in 1970, I treated along psychoanalytic lines a number of patients in private practice who had been or would have been diagnosed as schizophrenic. At the time, this was not necessarily the prevailing culture of the anti-psychiatry groups with which I was involved. R. D. Laing, who had been trained as a psychoanalyst in the British Society, and his colleagues were critical not only of psychiatrists but also of the "orthodoxy" of psychoanalysts. Nevertheless, I had come from a psychoanalytic tradition that taught me that psychoanalysis, unlike psychiatry, was not concerned with restraining or subduing madness. Therefore, there was no contradiction, in principle, between the questioning of psychiatry on the one hand and the clinical practice of psychoanalysis on the other.

Perhaps today, nearly six decades after *The Divided Self* (Laing, 1960) was first published, it is difficult to understand how innovative the shift suggested by Laing's work was for many contemporary clinicians in the United Kingdom. He considered the experience of the psychotic as a true experience, rather than as a falsified one. He did not doubt the immediate subjective experience of the psychotic; this never meant that the patient was not psychotic, nor that her psychosis should not be treated. Laing restored a sense of respect for all psychotic phenomena as something strange, alien, perhaps beyond interpretation. Like Freud many years earlier, he challenged clinicians to listen to patients, even to those who appeared hopelessly mad. The psychotic, in all of us, refers to something unknowable, elusive to any kind of certainty. At times, the analyst treating psychotic patients might glimpse this through an act of intuition, a gut reaction that results in "bursting out" with an inexplicable clinical intervention. Then, the analyst gets closer, in himself as much as in the patient, to something that otherwise remains unspoken, out of reach. Since psychosis might elude definition, Laing argued, it might not be accessible to any form of simplified psychological resolution.

Insanity is not just unreason, nor is it necessarily a failure of reason. Even if psychotic subjects do not know what to do with their knowledge, they may often have a disconcerting, accurate insight into their madness. This accounts for some rather inspired insights by psychotic patients, a self-conscious awareness that nevertheless produces so much suffering and deception of self and others.

Traditionally, if the clinical presentation of patients included hallucinations and delusions, a loss of capacity to relate to others, if they appeared to be detached, unresponsive, and negativistic, a diagnosis of schizophrenia was likely to be made. Even today, the diagnosis of schizophrenia seems to depend, at least partly, on the ideology and conception of illness held by the clinician. The symptoms mentioned above might, indeed, be indicative of such a condition, but not necessarily so. It is an unavoidable tragedy that sometimes such diagnoses can only be confirmed with the passing of time, when the progression of the illness brings about a deterioration of the subject's capacity for relatedness. Even this seems to be put in question by those cases of schizophrenia that present themselves as a series of acute episodes without the above-mentioned deterioration.

It is worth mentioning here, in this respect, a related diagnosis, that of *bouffées delirantes*, which is a concept that has been exclusively developed and used in France. It was traditionally closely associated with severe forms of hysteria and describes acute episodes characterised by the sudden eruption of a transitory psychosis that can last from a few weeks to a few months. The most important diagnostic aspect of the breakdown is its character of suddenness. Otherwise, it presents features very similar to a schizophrenic breakdown: numerous and exuberant hallucinations, paranoid ideas, sexual confusion, delusions of grandeur, and so forth. I often thought that Tony could have been diagnosed as suffering from this type of acute hallucinatory psychosis, which can sometimes be precipitated by the use of drugs (Ey, Bernard & Brisset, 1965).

It can be argued that a considerable number of the seriously ill patients described in the literature and seen in our consulting rooms might be disturbed hysterics after all. Perhaps the diagnosis of *hysterical psychosis* should be rescued (Libbrecht, 1995; Maleval, 1981). Plenty of patients would fit this clinical description; there are hysterical patients who are undoubtedly psychotic. Nevertheless, the structural reasons or theoretical justification required for placing hysteria among the psychoses would be highly questionable.

Bion established the important difference between psychotic and non-psychotic personalities coexisting within one subject. According to him, the difference between the two personalities depends on the splitting of everything that concerns awareness of internal and external reality and the expulsion into, or the engulfing of, objects (Bion, 1957). The preponderance of destructive impulses, being so intense in disturbed patients, turns their love impulses into sadism. There is a hatred of reality (a point originally made by Freud, 1924, p. 149), together with a dread of imminent annihilation. Bion also suggested that there is "a premature and precipitate formation of object relations, foremost amongst which is the transference, whose thinness is in marked contrast with the tenacity with which they are maintained. The prematurity, thinness and tenacity are pathognomonic" (p. 44). This seems to have been confirmed by many other clinicians. A patient who suffers from separation anxiety at the first weekend of the analysis – as if he had been coming for treatment for years – would lead me indeed to consider this reaction pathognomonic of serious borderline pathology (Kohon, 2007).

In the case of Tony, his psychotic personality seemed to coexist with his non-psychotic one in a way that allowed his ego not to be wholly withdrawn from reality. The non-psychotic personality was never obscured by the psychotic one. While the prematurity and the tenacity were certainly present in Tony's transference from the beginning, the thinness was not. His analysis was conducted for a long period of time under the dominance of an idealised transference, which remained mostly untouched. While this helped him to avoid further feelings of vulnerability (Rosenfeld, 1987), it also allowed him to express his true despair, his sense of being lost in the world, and his wish to be helped. This should not be seen as a technical suggestion equivalent to active encouragement through reassurance or expressions of love, nor as an attempt to provide a new and better parental figure in the analyst, who would "make up" for the environmental failures of the past.

At times, Tony had difficulties in believing that I existed; he was obviously relieved to see me at the following session. I thought that Tony hallucinated my existence: he created me through his desires. This could be something that disturbed patients need to do. To interpret it as a negative, regressive action would only interfere with the process of recovery. To encourage it through unnecessary so-called supportive interventions on the part of the analyst could be seductive and/or detrimental.

In stark contrast to Tony, Barbara presented an appearance of a seriously neurotic, perhaps rather perverse, certainly lost soul – but there was nothing "psychotic" as such in her. I did exist in her mind, but only in a profoundly eroticised manner. She could not fully comprehend, nor did she seem to want to understand, the disturbance of her psychic internal world and its consequences in her external world; she lived in permanent chaos, but her awareness of it was superficial. She wanted her anxieties to disappear, "just to be happy". She refused to be "a patient": the possibility of an experience of passivation in the treatment was inaccessible to her.[1]

There will always be an intense pressure exerted on the analyst by disturbed and perverse patients to give up the psychoanalytic setting. I always found it most useful, and certainly safest for both the patient and the analyst, to adhere to a psychoanalytic mode of working. This mode cannot and should not be rigid. Herbert Rosenfeld, Donald Winnicott, and Hanna Segal – three of the four leading British analysts (the other being Wilfred Bion) who promoted the treatment of psychotic patients using the essentials of the psychoanalytic technique – introduced changes in their analytic approach. Although Rosenfeld and Segal described these changes as "minor changes" and "minor deviations" (Rosenfeld, 1947, p. 311; Segal, 1957, p. 101), they can be seen, at least in the case of Winnicott and Rosenfeld, both of whom gave more details of their technique, as fairly substantial. For example, Rosenfeld did not ask schizophrenic patients to lie on the couch: many of them were "better treated in the sitting-up position" (1952, p. 65); he saw them at least six times a week; he did not take long breaks (not more than a few days) while treating patients in an acute state of psychosis; and, more importantly, he gave the patients "if necessary, longer sessions (90 minutes) while the acute phase persists" (1952, p. 66).

Given the confusion between thought and action on the part of disturbed patients, these measures might seem "minor" to the analyst, but they may not be so for the patient, who interprets them as non-verbal forms of reassurance and expressions of love. Winnicott says:

> For the neurotic, the couch and warmth and comfort can be *symbolical* of the mother's love; for the psychotic, it would be more true to say that these things are the analyst's expression of love. The couch is the analyst's lap or womb, and the warmth is the live warmth of the analyst's body. And so on.
>
> (Winnicott, 1947b, p. 199)

This certainly proved to have been the case with Tony.

I decided, after the second year of analysis, to change from the 90-minute sessions that I had been offering him up to then, following the example of Rosenfeld and other colleagues, like Enid Balint (personal communication, 1987), to the usual 50 minutes. I became aware that I did not want to offer him prolonged sessions any longer; I did not wish to treat him in any "special" way. Not surprisingly, Tony reacted with anger, resentment, and actual physical tantrums during the sessions. He refused to leave the room, claiming that he was not going to allow me to love other patients more than I loved him. It took time, hard work, and a lot of trust on his part for Tony to accept that it was not a matter of loving others more than him but that, even though he might have been the only patient I was seeing for prolonged sessions, I was choosing not to love him more than others.

The relevance of keeping a proper psychoanalytic setting becomes very important here. The regularity of the sessions, the reliability of the analyst, the attention given to the patient, the adherence to an interpretative mode, the working-through of psychic conflicts, all this offers the possibility for psychotic patients to make a slow, painful recovery. It is the consistency of the psychoanalytic setting that allows for what Winnicott called "moments of illusion" to occur:

> at the start, simple contact with external or shared reality has to be made, by the infant's hallucinating and the world's presenting, with moments of illusion for the infant in which the two are taken by him to be identical, which they never in fact are.
>
> (Winnicott, 1945, p. 154)

When Winnicott spoke of "moments of illusion", he was referring to the beginning of life, the moment of the encounter of mother and baby. By now, most of us have heard it many times: if it is true that there is no such thing as an infant without a mother, then it is also equally true that there is no such thing as a mother and baby without a father, imaginary or real. The analytic encounter itself cannot be understood in terms of just the mother-and-baby relationship. Mother and baby can only exist in the context of a third term, which does not need to be physically present in order to be there.

The third term, albeit not the only one, of all analyses, which regulates the relationship between patient and analyst, is defined and made present by the psychoanalytic setting. This notion was elaborated in the 1960s by Enrique Pichon-Rivière in his teachings. The importance of maintaining a proper setting, including whatever modifications the analyst might decide to introduce, can be better understood through the study that Bleger (a disciple of Pichon-Rivière) made of the psychoanalytic frame. He defined the frame as a permanent presence, a stable non-process. While the process is always variable, it constitutes the material of the sessions and can be studied, analysed, and interpreted; the frame forms the background of a unique Gestalt. The frame is a "dumb" institution defined by the psychoanalytic contract that establishes the formal terms of the arrangements agreed to by patient and analyst. It is always there, possibly used at times as a defence against psychotic anxiety, similarly to the way in which we tend to use institutions (Jaques, 1955), or as a depository of the psychotic part of the personality (Bleger, 1967). Bleger described it as the "most primitive and undifferentiated organisation", never noticed unless it is missing, which receives the projection of the patient's "ghost world".

The psychoanalytic frame helps patient and analyst know that whatever else is going on in the analysis, the analysis continues. The frame exists in the mind of the analyst, and it is up to him to preserve it, trust in it, have the ability to use it. The existence and preservation of this frame, and the analyst's own basic trust in the psychoanalytic process, are the conditions for the moments of illusion to be created. The analytic frame also has the function of protecting the patient during the course of the analysis, in comparable fashion to the mother's role as a protective shield during the child's development (Khan, 1963). If during a long analysis there were to be breaches and failures of the frame, these can produce a cumulative trauma, which develops in silent and invisible ways but which nevertheless acquires the value of trauma, if only in retrospect. Many instances of analytic impasse (as described by Rosenfeld, 1987) could be the result, as much as the proof, of the presence of this cumulative process.[2]

While Barbara could not fully accept the terms of the psychoanalytic contract, to settle, accept, and be contained by the psychoanalytic situation, Tony used the psychoanalytic frame as a very effective depository of the psychotic part of his personality. At the beginning of his treatment, Tony's fate appeared to be sealed; he was paralysed in time and seemed destined to remain forever self-institutionalised. A certain degree of self-institutionalisation is part of any normal development. In growing up, the human subject is by necessity unconsciously forced, in different circumstances and with a variety of intensities, to surrender to the other's desire; it is part of a developmental process of learning by which the individual becomes a social being. The environment imposes this learning on the subject, who gives up or tones down his unconscious desires for the price of survival, acceptance, and recognition (Castoriadis, 1997; see also Balibar, 1994; Fryer, 2004). A process of de-subjectivation allows subjectivity to develop. However, self-institutionalisation should never be fully achieved or completed, otherwise one would witness the triumph of the death instinct at the service of the Other.[3]

The subject has to remain free to recreate meaning, to be unpredictable, to surprise himself and others through his actions. The alternative is to inhabit a self that functions like a protective institution; like a jail or a hospital, a family or a neighbourhood, the institutionalised self becomes a safe refuge that the fading subject is unwilling to leave. There are two basic fears that determine this process. One is the fear of change; the other is the fear of attack (Pichon-Rivière, 1967). These fears make the subject reluctant to move away from an emotional status quo already achieved, refusing to face any new situation. This process can progressively become a tragic and pathological cul-de-sac, a passive adaptation to a reality that is experienced as menacing and hostile (Kohon, 1999). A depressive apathy towards any possibility of change can ensue: there is a lack of initiative, together with a loss of interest in the outside world.

There is a malignant passivity that makes some patients appear submissive to others, but the only safe place they can find is their very illness. These subjects develop a way of being in the world that, through sterile repetition, falsely promises a personal safety net. Through a destructive element embedded in their persistence in being, their illness may remain relatively contained within their rigid measures of psychic safety; we might only learn about their madness through their acting out in the process of treatment – hence the value of such acting out in psychoanalysis. On the other hand, in obsessional patients, for example, the madness will be expressed only in their compulsive thoughts; this confinement might help to keep them sane, for the madness is limited to one area, keeping the rest of their personality fairly safe.

In the process of becoming a subject, we are inevitably at the mercy of external events over which we have no control. Nevertheless, we have to make our choices, decide our destiny. This is one reason why Freud spoke of a "choice of neurosis", a concept that, however apparently mysterious, confronts the problem of why and how a person may fall ill (1915b, p. 317). Freud implied through this concept that the subject actively, though unconsciously, participates in the illness. Only then, once the historical and constitutional determinants of the illness are assumed by the subject as a choice, do they become meaningful and "attain the force of motivating factors" (Laplanche & Pontalis, 1967). The same is implied in the Freudian concept of object-choice, a choice far removed from being a mere intellectual act. The subject's actions are determined by his unconscious, but that does not make him less responsible for them. "Tragedy means, above all else", says Alford, "that people are responsible without being free" (1992, p. 115). Oedipus' fate was overdetermined, thus not free, but he took symbolic responsibility for his actions when he declared that, although many of his sufferings were the work of Apollo, it was his own choice, carried out by his own hand, to blind himself. Freud's view in this regard is best illustrated by his appealing to an Austrian law when, in response to the Rat Man's objections to his interpretations, he said that

> it is well known, of course, that it was equally punishable to say, "The Emperor is an ass" or to disguise the forbidden words by saying "If anyone says, etc. ... then he will have me reckon with."
>
> (Freud, 1909, p. 179)

Winnicott seemed to have understood that madness is the most personal characteristic of a human being. In order to feel alive, to experience passion and be creative, a subject has to accept that he will be "forever caught in a conflict, nicely balanced between the fear of madness and the need to be mad" (1965, p. 126).

Paradox is the nature of the beast, the very subject of psychoanalytic inquiry.

Notes

1 The passivation of the baby in relation to the mother was described by Green (1980): it involves the baby needing to "submit" to the care provided by the mother; the baby has to trust that the mother will not take advantage of his/her vulnerability; that the mother will not misunderstand his/her "language".

2 Enrique Pichon-Rivière and José Bleger were two of the most important and influential figures in the history of psychoanalysis in Argentina. Inspired by Pichon-Rivière, Bleger's thoughts concerning the psychoanalytic frame were central to my psychoanalytic education while still a psychology student at university, where he was one of my teachers. Decades later, Bleger's (1967) paper on the subject has become an important contribution, internationally recognised, to the theory and technique of psychoanalysis. According to PEP-Web,

British psychoanalytic authors who have recently referred to this particular aspect of his work include: Robin Anderson (2017); Catalina Bronstein (2014); Penelope Crick (2014); Alessandra Lemma (2014); Rosine Perelberg (2007); John Steiner (2013).

3 At a socio-political level, tyrannical, totalitarian, repressive governments attempt – and at times unfortunately succeed in – imposing extreme forms of de-subjectivation on their citizens. In Western democratic countries, there is growing uneasiness about the restrictions and controls imposed by political leaders and government figures, such measures being justified through rationalised versions of an over-protective pseudo-concern – the product of the so-called "nanny state".

5

THE HEROIC ACHIEVEMENT OF SANITY

Given the fact that human beings are born prematurely, compared to other higher mammals, they only survive thanks to the intervention of a physical and psychological environment that will protect them, look after them, feed them, and in general terms help them to develop for a relatively long time. Freud described the human baby as being born in a state of helplessness, with no capacity to help itself. The baby is completely dependent on other people for the satisfaction of its most basic needs. The parental or care-giving environment can be said to fulfil the function, in the outside world, of a protective shield (Khan, 1963).

Freud believed that there were two types of helplessness at this initial stage in life: motor helplessness, in reference to the specific action that is needed to satisfy a need, and psychic helplessness, the inability of the psychic apparatus to cope with and control the increase in tension. While, in *Beyond the Pleasure Principle* (1920a), Freud saw as traumatic "any situations from outside which are powerful enough to break through the protective shield" (p. 29), in *Inhibitions, Symptoms and Anxiety* (1926a), helplessness became the prototype of the traumatic situation.

According to Laplanche and Pontalis, the concept of helplessness "is at the root of several lines of psycho-analytic inquiry"; it is at the core of the vicissitudes of human relationships and the understanding of trauma (Kohon, 2005, 2007, 2016, 2018; see also, Perelberg, 2015, 2018). From the genetic point of view,

> it is on the basis of this idea that we are able to understand the primordial role played by the experience of satisfaction, its

hallucinatory reproduction and the distinction between the primary and secondary processes.

(Laplanche & Pontalis, 1967, p. 190)

The importance of this first experience of satisfaction, which will determine all future experiences of pleasure, resides in the fact that the hallucinatory process does not deny reality. Just the opposite: it helps to recognise the existence of a reality outside the self, different from it, which needs to be found. The hallucinatory process helps the baby to recognise such a thing as a breast, existing in the world as part of a mother. More than anything else, it shows the baby's wish to take possession of the breast inside his mouth. We can imagine here a structural state of primary narcissism, where all wishes are fulfilled through omnipotence and hallucination.

At the same time, if the baby is not omnipotent, then someone else has to be, in order to save the baby from total destruction: "the state of helplessness [of the baby] implies the mother's omnipotence" (Laplanche & Pontalis, 1967, p. 190); this omnipotence is projected onto the object. Furthermore, it is plausible that once the baby is confronted with the fact that the mother does not provide absolutely everything, all the time, the baby begins to achieve a sense of reality; object relatedness progressively replaces primary megalomania and grandiosity. In Winnicott's terms, the mother's gradual failings and the recognition of her existence independently of the baby's omnipotence will create the possibility for the infant to move onto the next stage, that of "relative dependence" (Winnicott, 1960b, p. 60).

Since the primary objects represent everything that is powerful and desirable, the child will identify and internalise these idealised objects; magically, one could argue, the baby would want to become mother and father. These identifications with, and internalisations of, the idealised parental objects serve as "models" for the subject. Inevitably, these models will never completely replace the omnipotent ideal of lost perfection. Thus, the subject's ego will always try to fill the gap between its own reality and its ideal, narcissistic longing for a (re-)union with the primary object. Unrealistic wishes and ambitions give way to achievable aims, but the ego ideal never gives up its magical qualities; grandiose values are never relinquished.

Given the total dependence of the human infant on its environment, how could the mother not be omnipotent? First, she is the one who has given birth to the baby; then, she makes it possible for the baby to survive; and, finally, she is the provider of the original experiences of safety and of pleasure. This omnipotent mother, who can do anything, does not need anyone else. The fixation on this relationship with a primary object, in the initial phase of an exclusive as well as intense lasting attachment, will be the source of psychotic states and perversions – and at the origin of all forms of love.

The inevitable discrepancy between the baby's helplessness and the mother's omnipotence prepares the ground for the possibility of primary violence:

> the mother's discourse ... is the agent responsible for the effect of anticipation imposed on the infant, from whom a response is expected that it is not in his power to give.
>
> (Aulagnier, 1975, p. 11)

Physical dependence on others for survival goes hand in hand with emotional immaturity; babies are at the mercy of potentially overwhelming anxieties and frustrations. The mother imposes her desire on the baby by, for example, offering and pushing her nipple into the baby's mouth. This could, in certain circumstances, reinforce the sense of helplessness in the baby. But, as Freud, Winnicott, Klein, and others have shown, the baby is far from passive. Melanie Klein has given us an insightful description of the baby's active searching, not so much for an object but for what could be defined as the pleasure of the object (Green, 2002). The breast is the infant's first object of desire, the mother, the first object of love. The physical relationship with mother (nursing, touching, being cuddled and caressed) necessarily includes sexual and erotic feelings. Klein stated it thus:

> I would not assume that the breast is [to the baby] merely a physical object. The whole of his instinctual desires and his unconscious phantasies imbue the breast with qualities going far beyond the actual nourishment it affords.
>
> (Klein, 1957, p. 180)

It is not only the baby who invests the breast with such qualities and wishes. From the beginning of life, it takes – at least – two to tango. What is on offer is not just milk; it also includes the mother's own instinctual desires and unconscious phantasies. In this encounter between two unconsciouses, the breast is a libidinal object for both participants; the dynamics of give-and-take are multidimensional and overdetermined. The baby is confronted with the task of metabolising something that never presents itself as always the same: he will never know quite what he will get next time round. Warm milk, cold milk, milk that tastes sour, poisonous milk, milk too rich to be comfortably digested, milk received from an eroticised breast, milk that gives pleasure, the same milk, inaugurating a life of un-pleasure: not just milk, then, not just simple nourishment to help him survive, but a complex emotional package to be unwrapped and metabolised. So, here it is: the first mouthful of meaning that the baby will receive. Love and hate: the scene in which the drama of love is staged originates in need, and at this point the fear of the loss of love is equivalent to the fear of not being able to survive.

The stage of dependence lasts for a long time, creating the conditions for a fruitful process of learning. From the first experience of feeding, some sort of pattern will be established; if the experiences are frequent and good enough, there will a representation of the "breast". The baby will be able to desire and represent the breast that he needs for his survival. Whenever the breast re-appears, fulfilling the desire of the subject, love is possible. Nevertheless, the good breast is never just good: the appearance itself of desire denotes the absence of what is missing. The relationship with the breast entails the ongoing process of comings and goings, of the mother's presence and absence. With each absence, if it is not too prolonged, the desire for her presence is established more clearly.

The search for an object in the real world is governed entirely by a relationship to signs. The dynamics of the *Fort–Da*, through the symbolic representation of the presence and absence of the mother, portrays the mythical moment of the acquisition of language. The unconscious might not be structured like a language, but language plays a fundamental and decisive part in the establishment and structuring of the baby's subjectivity. From the beginning of life, the subject relates to other subjects.[1] Even before he has developed his capacity for linguistic expression – one could argue, even before birth – he lives in a cultural milieu that provides a context for and extensive references to his existence. We are conceived, born, and exist in a world of others: it is these relationships that give meaning to our lives. These subjects are desiring subjects, who impose their own linguistic code on the newcomer. The baby arrives in a meaningful world, marked and defined by language. The baby is born in a human world of enigmatic signifiers (Laplanche, 1987) that are alien to him. There is an unconscious process of implantation of enigmatic verbal and non-verbal messages in the primitive body-ego of the infant, messages derived from the adults' sexuality. Laplanche describes this as the *fundamental anthropological situation* of the human infant. Being enigmatic, these signifiers are the source of innumerable misunderstandings. The baby falls into a world of significant others: mother, father, grandparents, with their own desires and their histories, their dreams and their own personal myths. The baby is to discover that, prior to his birth, he has been existing in the mind of others; he has been given a name, has become part of a myth determined by others' desires. The world that welcomes him belongs to others; there will always be a considerable plus of signification that the baby will not be able to decode.

In a scene described by A. S. Byatt in her novel *Still Life*, a mother is talking to her newborn son: "She had not expected ecstasy. She noted that he was both much more solid, and, in the feebleness of his fluttering movements of lip and cheek muscle, the dangerous lolling of his uncontrolled head, more fragile, than she had expected." (Byatt, 1985, p. 100). The mother puts out a finger and touches the baby's fist. Following a primitive instinct, the baby curls his tiny fingers round the mother's own, clutching it, loosening it, tightening again. "'There', she said to him, and he looked, and the light poured through the window, brighter and brighter, and his eyes saw it, and hers, and she was aware of bliss, a word she didn't like, the only one" (p. 101). There *she* was: her body, quiet; her mind, free and clear. There *he* was: the boy and his eyes, but seeing what? "The boy would change. But now in the sun she recognised him, and recognised that she did not know, and had never seen him, and loved him, in the bright new air with a simplicity she had never expected to know. 'You', she said to him, skin for the first time on skin in the outside air, which was warm and shining, 'you'" (p. 101).

The mother gives meaning to the baby's experiences, a meaning that the baby cannot yet create by himself. The mother anticipates what the baby is due to discover. When the mother speaks, she inaugurates a dialogue, an exchange between herself and her baby, that is unique and fundamental. While the mother uses language, mother and baby operate within a proto-linguistic system (Bruner, 1990), communicating with each other. The constitution of the baby's subjectivity is realised through a series of consecutive and dialectical representations and misrepresentations of this original primary scenario in which mother and baby interact. It is these words – *"there", "you"* – as we imagine them being spoken with love by the mother, that make the subjectivity of the baby possible. "You", says she, the giver of meaning, provider of goodness, source of contentment. How does the baby interpret this declaration of love? The word of the mother, if spoken with pleasure, will create pleasure. If uttered with love, it will be assimilated as part of the self and generate love. But if the word is not there, or the voice is hateful, uncertain, or troubled by too much ambivalence, if it is misleading or deceitful, then the baby responds with confusion, insecurity, and a sense of loss. The word of the significant other will remain in this case an alien object, a separate internal object that will become persecuting, attacking the creative possibilities of integration and links. Pleasure will be replaced by uncertainty, love substituted with fear. Excessive love, or exclusive love offered by an omnipotent giver, will determine an anxious response.

This has been described in Lacan's reformulation of the mirror stage in his *Seminars* (1960–61). In his revised view, the parent, holding the child up to the mirror, offers a verbal gesture of approval; the image offered by the mirror is internalised and libidinally invested by the infant, confirming the child's existence as a whole. We have a significant scenario here: the parent's recognition of the child in the mirror is what becomes truly important. The child is not, after all, the one celebrating on his own the discovery of his specular image in a mythical moment of narcissistic jubilation (as originally described by Lacan, 1936 [1949]). The parent, or parental figures, saying "you, you, that is you" offer the necessary recognition and acknowledgement. The other-than-himself of the mirror is pulled away, forced either to look at the mother or at least listen to the mother. The intervention of a linguistic code establishes the presence of a third term, right from birth.

For different theoretical reasons, Lacan, as well as Melanie Klein, both postulated a precocious Oedipus complex. Lacan called it *le toujours-déjà-là*, the always-already-there of the complex. There is no pre-oedipal without an oedipal structure; in fact, that is why it is called pre-oedipal; the oedipal is there, if only as a negative reference. If the visual were the only origin of subjectivity, the subject would then be trapped in a narcissistic predicament. But the word of the mother introduces a break in the process of primary identification of the baby with his narcissistic image in the mirror. The words of this pre-oedipal mother represent the confirmation that she constitutes herself as a primitive third term in the baby's mind. This is a true dialectical moment: the recognition of the subjectivity of the baby through the signifying utterances of the mother denotes – implies – the simultaneous recognition of her own subjectivity. The progressive development of these subjectivities and their mutual recognition reduces the mother's omnipotence and the baby's need to use extreme defences. It inaugurates an inter-subjective space, a transitional space that is at the core of the process of symbolisation.

The two aspects of the original state of helplessness – the hallucinatory experience of satisfaction on the one hand, and the omnipotence of the mother on the other – create the conditions for a normal madness to develop. This madness is only tempered by the presence of a third term in the mind of the mother. This is the time when what will be on offer to the baby dangerously borders on excess: presence and absence, love and hate, attention and indifference, closeness and distance, physical contact and avoidance; all of this can be too much. Or too soon. Or too little. Or too late. In fact, this normal madness is none other than the world of internal objects as described by Klein: primitive fears and terrors and intense and extreme anxieties. In her early view, initial object relations were shaped by very sadistic phantasies; in her mature view, she understood the earliest phantasy life of the infant in terms of equal extremes of love and hate in which very good and very bad objects coexisted and had to be kept apart. Klein's compelling description of the baby's internal world does not exclude exposure to a natural, unavoidable, and yet potentially traumatic imposition from the outside.

André Green called this situation "original madness" ("maternal madness", in the French version) (Green, 1980; see also Eigen, 1999). It is, indeed, original: it takes place at the origins of normal individual human development, at the peak of intense primitive psychic activity. It is also original in the sense of its uniqueness: it represents something "absolutely personal" for the individual, being at the core of who she is (Winnicott, 1965). It is the personal madness present later in all forms of love, clearly visible in transference-love. It is there in all manifestations of the drives, in every expression of sexuality; it is the madness of pleasure and desire, of narcissism and idealisation, a basic madness that informs human life right from the start.

I would prefer to call this madness "normal", in Winnicott's sense: "Normal is what is there", he said (1970, p. 270). The baby does not know anything else; the use of extreme primary defences at the onset of life is nothing but justified. The baby gets what he can, and, if he wants to survive – and one assumes that most babies do – then he might have to take whatever he gets, in whatever way he can. If the emotional nourishment on offer is toxic or poisoned, contaminated by hate, envy, jealousy, and so on, then extreme measures and counter-attacks might be necessary and be called upon to digest it (Eigen, 1999). It makes perfect, "normal" sense. Thus understood, madness is not an occasional alteration in adult mental life; it is an inevitable component of psychic life throughout the subject's life, as long as she continues to experience emotions and is capable of passion. First experienced in the initial encounter with mother, it will be at the core of the subject's unconscious. Like the residues of a dream, it will reappear, more or less in disguise, in every aspect of the subject's internal life. At the origin, it can be argued, there was madness – sanity is a surplus benefit (J. Sekoff, personal communication, 2000), not included in the initial bargain of being born. Sanity is the result of a process whereby the use and the impact of primitive defences slowly decreases. Subjectivity and relative neurotic normality appear as genuinely heroic achievements (Eigen, 1999).

Early normal madness does not necessarily create psychosis. Green introduced a distinction between madness and psychosis. Madness is not pathological; it is linked to "the vicissitudes of a primordial Eros" (Green, 1980). In fact, this follows the *Oxford English Dictionary*'s definition of these two words. While psychosis, in modern times, describes any mental illness accompanied by hallucinations, delusions, mental confusion, and/or loss of contact with reality, madness is a more inclusive concept: it describes a multiplicity of phenomena, from insanity to rage, anger, or violence. To be mad could cover being stupefied by fear or suffering; being carried away by enthusiasm or desire; to be infatuated; wildly excited, extravagant (*Oxford English Dictionary*).

Piera Aulagnier (1975) speaks of a psychotic potentiality in the baby, a madness that in normal circumstances can be contained within the relationship with the mother. Sometimes such containment fails to happen. In his description of the fundamental anthropological situation of the human infant, Laplanche introduced the concept of intromission, a "violent variant" of the normal process of implantation. In the case of intromission, the message is not allowed to be decoded; the violence of the parents in sending the message actively interferes with the possibility of translation and metabolisation. It is not just that these tasks are difficult by definition, but that the infant is subjected to a malignant process that "puts into the interior an element resistant to all metabolisation" (Laplanche, 1956, p. 136). Implantation can turn into intromission for a variety of reasons. For example, the existence of unknown constitutional factors might determine a weak primitive body-ego (Freud, 1923, p. 26) that does not provide enough of a protective shield against the messages received. Also, mothering functions might be repeated and prolonged for too long; they might be unduly intense or emotionally charged in such a way that the actions change their meaning. Unknown and/or unpredicted factors might also contribute to the failure of translation, producing unsuccessful attempts at metabolising signifiers. Finally, another important factor might be the presence of an intense, unbound sexuality that permeates and contaminates every action on the part of the adult.

If the mother's response to the baby's needs is inadequate, the baby tends to organise his responses in a distorted fashion. From clinical experience we can tentatively conclude that, given certain circumstances, madness develops into proper psychosis whenever a baby, in the throes of having to cope with his own madness, has to deal with the madness of the primary object as well. If this is too frequent and too intense, it becomes a cumulative trauma (Khan, 1963): a malignant pattern is progressively established. A deluded, depressed, pathologically disturbed mother is not able to contain her baby's projections, anxieties, and feelings. Her anxious response to the excesses of love and hate of that primary relationship intensify, rather than minimise, the baby's own responses. In psychosis, what has not been repressed in the parents returns as delusions in the psychosis of their child (Aulagnier, 1975). As delusions, they reveal in a distorted manner what had originally failed to be repressed in the parents but which by now cannot be identified. At its worst, this might constitute the beginning of a truly delusional process. From the original situation of normal madness, the relationship might develop into a shared love/hate psychosis between mother and baby. Ironically, a psychotic pact might help the mother to sustain an apparent sanity; it acts as scaffolding that prevents the collapse of the building.

Normal madness makes its most dramatic and undeniable reappearance in the situation of transference. Strange love this, the patient's transference-love towards a stranger. Analysis creates the conditions for this love to develop, greatly helped by the intense resistance that announces that the subject prefers to repeat rather than remember. This intriguing piece of real life erupting into the consulting room with uncanny strength cannot be ignored, dismissed, or reduced to a compulsion to repeat repressed infantile conflicts. As distressing and, at times, comical as the situation of an intense and passionate transference-love may be, it is also serious (Freud, 1915a, p. 159). Things to do with love, like transference, cannot be compared to any other emotional phenomena, "they are … written on a special page on which no other writing is tolerated" (p. 160). But transference-love, this "spirit of the underworld" that we have summoned up "by cunning spells" (p. 164), is it real? Is it true?

Freud's summary is worth quoting at length:

> We have no right to dispute that the state of being in love which makes its appearance in the course of analytic treatment has the character of a "genuine" love. If it seems so lacking in normality, this is sufficiently explained by the fact that being in love in ordinary life, outside analysis, is also more similar to abnormal than to normal mental phenomena. Nevertheless, transference-love is characterized by certain features which ensure it a special position. In the first place, it is provoked by the analytic situation; secondly, it is greatly intensified by the resistance, which dominates the situation; and thirdly, it is lacking to a high degree in a regard for reality, is less sensible, less concerned about the consequence and more blind in its valuation of the loved person than we are prepared to admit in the case of normal love. We should not forget, however, that *these departures from the norm constitute precisely what is essential about being in love.*
>
> (Freud, 1915a, pp. 168–169; italics added)

As experiences go, transference, always related to an object in the present, has an unparalleled immediacy. Nevertheless, no psychoanalytic situation can be reduced to, and/or limited to, its interpretation. Some psychoanalysts indeed suffer from the fascination of continuously decoding the content of what is being said by the patient in terms of the transference, creating the illusion of a thorough understanding, behaving as though "transference" equals "the unconscious". Transference interpretations create a meaning of sorts, but they do not constitute the meaning of all meanings.

Most of the time, in the treatment of psychotic and seriously borderline patients, we are dealing with something unspeakable. If the unconscious were structured like a language, treatment of these patients would be impossible. Even taking into consideration the uncertainty of these cures, they show that psychoanalysis, though unable to go beyond language, is still capable of cutting across it. In most cases, psychotic patients live in a constant state of psychic agony, which is not only unthinkable (Winnicott, 1963 [1974]) but also unnameable. In the analysis, they move from intense separation anxiety to the terror of being intruded upon by the analyst's presence and words. While they develop a passionate attachment to the analyst and to the sessions, the horror of being intruded upon is always threatening the relationship with the analyst. This is at the core of the fear of further breakdowns. How can the analyst help the patient to make this agony bearable?

The main difficulty resides in the patient's central dilemma: needing the analysis, on the one hand, but, on the other, experiencing the psychoanalytic situation itself as a repetition of the original trauma. The patient might want and need the analyst's words but tries to avoid them; the need itself is experienced as a great humiliation. The analyst, in trying to make sense of the patient's predicament, re-enacts a trauma that perhaps could not even have been experienced in the past (Winnicott, 1954). In many cases, the communication with the patient becomes itself traumatic (Kohon, 1999). The presence as well as the absence of the analyst is experienced as impingement. For the infant, events in life are experienced as impingement when the infant is not able to process what is happening to him (Winnicott, 1949 [1954], 1962). Instead of being able to digest the experience and use it for growth and further development, the infant reacts with panic and terror. A mismatch has occurred between the baby and the environment. Confusion between love and hate ensues, and this makes it impossible for the subject to discriminate between good and bad objects.

Rosenfeld described patients feeling phobic about their own mothers: they are terrified that they have to defend themselves against something extremely dangerous – as when, for example, the physical experience of being fed becomes confused with being poisoned (Rosenfeld, 1987). In analysis, the desire to be recognised by the analyst makes these patients feel vulnerable and eventually confused. To love and be loved come at a price. But such patients believe they will lose the precarious sense of reality that they have achieved so painfully and are convinced that they will have to replace their reality with the analyst's own version of it. Some of these patients do not seem to possess the necessary protective shield that would safeguard them from the outside world.

A subject, in order to remain sane, or to be saved from psychosis, needs somebody, an Other who can offer proof of "a certain complicity and closeness with the subject's thoughts and theories" (Aulagnier, 1975, p. 168). The French word, *complicité*, has to be properly understood. In French, as well as in Spanish, it refers to a close understanding between people. The nature of this *complicité* is clear: it is a way of letting the psychotic patient know that one is on her side. There is a commitment on the part of the analyst that needs to be made explicit, even if not actually spoken; the wish to help cannot be denied, hidden, or fudged.

Complicité and emotional closeness are sometimes manifested in the relationship with disturbed patients through the use of humour. Tony, for example, even though he was suffering from the horror of being paralysed in an emotional trap where life could feel inconceivable and death the only alternative, saved himself by having a strong sense of humour, which, although black and surrealistic, contained an expression of hope. Humour, at some stages of his treatment, constituted "the currency of intimacy" (Cohen, 1999) between us. In a true dialectical way, humour actually created and established this intimacy, which, I suspect, made Tony trust that he did not need to explain everything to me, nor did I have to spell out every interpretation to him. To quote Cohen's book on jokes:

> When we laugh at the same thing, that is a very special occasion. It is already noteworthy that we laugh at all, at anything, and that we laugh all alone. That we do it together is the satisfaction of a deep human longing, the realization of a desperate

> hope. It is the hope that we are enough like one another to sense one another, to be able to live together.
>
> (Cohen, 1999, p. 29)

The analyst might be scared by the passionate involvement of the patient who wants to be loved unconditionally – but has to accept the risk. This does not, by itself, compromise the psychoanalytic attitude and the professional boundaries demanded and required from an analyst. When the madness of the patient's love borders on psychosis, this is not only frightening for the analyst, it is also exhausting. The analyst is forced to fight a war against the patient's destructiveness, negative therapeutic reactions, repeated splitting, acting out. The intensity of the transference created by the "diabolical device of the Viennese doctor" (Kristeva, 1983, p. 9) can be extraordinary. Can we conceive of an analysis without transference, without the love generated by transference? Love is at the centre of transference, making all frustrations (including the sexual ones) bearable to the patient. It is *Liebe*, true libido, that helps the subject to open up his self to another subject and form a relationship with him. The sexual, never separated from love, never forgotten even if repressed, will be there. The patient might ask to be loved by the analyst at all costs, at times asking for a mutual pact of negation of reality.

Frequently, masochism occupies central stage: "Seduce me, please abuse me, do with me whatever you like, I want to prove my love to you" demands the patient, translating his original need for survival into a traumatic need for love and recognition (Kohon, 2005, p. 78). It can be argued that there is a "perverse" side to the analytic contract: one subject imposes on another certain conditions that, if accepted, enable the relationship to take place. The patient is supposed to relate every possible sexual fantasy, every dream, the details of intimate relationships to the analyst, who refuses to say much at all about himself! A power game? It can develop into one. However, in principle, the analyst's ethical commitment consists of refusing the position of power altogether in the first place.

As in a caricature, where certain normal features of a person are exaggerated and yet remain recognisable, here one can see the risks of the analytic enterprise with psychotic patients: they do not want to accept reality, the separation between self and others, between them and the analyst. They also refuse to acknowledge the differentiation of sexes or the generational conflict; they experience total love for an omnipotent, idealised object. The "as if" of the analytic encounter may be lost and denied for most of the initial, psychotic period of treatment; instead, they harbour the impossible hope that the analyst could be everything for them, forever.

I would agree with Herbert Rosenfeld's view regarding the need to assess carefully the patient's vulnerability and defensiveness (Rosenfeld, 1987). The idealisation of the analyst might be the only experience of love available to the patient; the analyst's attempts at interpreting the idealised transference could provoke a detrimental increase in the patient's envy and unnecessary experiences of humiliation. This demands a prudent and watchful consideration by the analyst of his countertransference; the patient's needs might be confused with the analyst's own neurotic desires. The narcissistic needs of the analyst can easily prolong the period of transference idealisation. And yet,

> It is important not to interfere with a patient's idealization of the analyst *just on principle*. A patient may have to make considerable progress in the analysis before he can accept the ups and downs of the analytic relationship, the battles which have to be fought, and the despair and emptiness which often seem unbearable.
>
> (Rosenfeld, 1987, p. 271; italics added)

Although he was strongly criticised, and his ideas not given serious weight by some of his Kleinian colleagues at the time of the publication of his book, I find Rosenfeld's clinical stance in this respect not only accurate but courageous. It is, no doubt, a complex and difficult question as to whether and when to interpret or not interpret the idealised transference. This is, after all, a clinical decision, taken by the analyst after careful consideration of the patient's vulnerability and of the analyst's own narcissistic needs. This is easier said than done. The analyst's clinical judgement is constantly at risk of being misled by the dynamics of projections and introjections taking place in the analytic encounter.

I would not suggest that the analyst should never interpret the idealised transference, only that this can wait, can be postponed. One of the main tasks of the analyst is to receive the patient's projective identifications (Money-Kyrle, 1956); this necessarily implies the need to accept them and contain them. There is plenty of time in an analysis to interpret those projections at the appropriate moment. In the analysis of Tony, I found that the idealised transference coexisted with, and perhaps even facilitated, the intensely negative feelings sometimes expressed in the letters he wrote to me. One set of feelings did not exclude the other.

No subject can assume that she is capable of love. To be able to love is as uncertain as to know with certainty that one is lovable. Disturbed patients can experience an intense sense of shame and unbearable pain when they find, in the process of an analysis, that their capacity for love is greatly diminished. It can throw them into further desolation and hopelessness. Envy and destructiveness can be made worse by their desperate need for help. Their experience of vulnerability, and feeling at the mercy of the analyst's designs, may increase the murderous attacks of their internal objects; this, in turn, makes the relationship with the analyst fraught with danger.

If patient and analyst have a therapeutic relationship over a long period of time, each becomes an inevitable witness to changes in the other. I cannot account for the way that Tony saw me and my practice change over the years. I am aware that he was particularly sensitive to all changes, including the variations of my mood, the way that I would phrase a question, or my tone of voice when I made an interpretation. The importance of these things in the treatment of disturbed patients has often been noted. On the other hand, in the psychoanalytic literature and in clinical presentations there has been a certain reluctance to admit how much liking or not liking the patient affects the therapeutic factors of an analysis. While it is not a necessary condition, liking a patient might play an important part in the treatment of patients. This is not to say that by itself it will help; nevertheless, it might, for example, affect the analyst's level of tolerance for the patient's regressive behaviour and destructiveness.

This presents a serious dilemma for the psychoanalyst treating patients originally identified by Rosenfeld as "thick-skinned", characterised by their insensitivity to deeper feelings (Rosenfeld, 1987). These are patients who are especially capable of provoking rejection in the analyst through their attempts at devaluing any form of help. In these cases, it might be difficult to discriminate between (a) a proper countertransference reaction (which can potentially be understood, contained, and eventually "given back" to the patient through interpretations); and (b) a genuine dislike that inhibits understanding. Ideally, we should be able to distinguish a response to the patient's transference from the analyst's inevitable transference to the patient.

Money-Kyrle's article on "normal countertransference" (1956) remains an inspiring source of further speculation and critical thought. He spoke in terms of both the analyst's reparative drives and the parental drives as complements to Freud's concept of "benevolent neutrality". I would say that countertransference could never be properly qualified as "normal", nor could it be associated with an attitude of "benevolent neutrality". As far as neutrality is concerned, the dictionary speaks of it as a state of "not supporting or helping either side in a conflict or disagreement", a state of impartiality. This refers to politics and wars, not to relationships. Neutrality, in psychoanalysis, applies to the analyst not taking active sides in conflicts or disagreements between the patient and others, outside the clinical situation; this is not always achieved. The dictionary also refers to the absence of "decided views or the expression of strong feelings". This needs further qualification: the analyst and his unconscious are too involved in the analytic relationship for either of these two alternatives not to occur. Both "decided views" and "strong feelings" will be felt, considered, and expressed, at some point or other, during the process of any analytic treatment.

Countertransference is, after all, a form of transference. It is always present and experienced by the analyst; it needs to be monitored, controlled, and yet also actively used by the analyst as a source of clinical data in the analytic session. The use of it will greatly depend on the analyst's training, experience, integrity, and ethical professional commitment; it requires a combined attitude of attentive caring, discretion, and prudence, together with an unobtrusive toughness to confront whatever might be necessary concerning the analytic relationship.

Ron Britton proposed the notion of an "ordinary positive countertransference", comparable to "the love of parents for children" (2003. p. 55). However, "parental love" is not "ordinary", nor can it be taken for granted – and, above all, it would never be just "positive". In any case, the relationship between parents and their children is not an accurate or unambiguous enough model to compare it to the relationship between analysts and their patients.

Given the often violent intensity of the analyst's countertransference reactions in the analysis of psychotic patients, liking or not liking a patient could be a decisive factor in their treatment. If this is accepted as an analytic parameter, the analyst is better able to deal with phenomena like hate in the countertransference. The analyst constantly moves from the maternal to the paternal position in the analysis of psychotic patients. He can never quite rest in one place and is always challenged to make urgent clinical decisions: either he offers a holding that makes the patient feel gratified and contained, or he establishes boundaries and differences (a handling) through the provisional meaning offered by his interpretations. In both cases, the analyst's aim is to promote the creation of a psychic space, even though this space is formed through the vicissitudes of an impossible and inevitably idealised love.

Freud declared that "the cure is effected by love" (Freud, 1906, pp. 12–13). The list of psychoanalytic authors who seemed to have misread, forgotten, misinterpreted, or distorted what Freud actually said is too long to be quoted. In fact, Freud, in his letter to Jung on 6 December 1906, was referring to "the fixation of the libido prevailing in the unconscious (transference)" (Freud, 1906, p. 12): in other words, he was clearly talking here about the transference-love of the analysand and not about the libidinal effects of the analyst's presence or actions. Love of the analyst is not the curative force in the treatment. While the patient will be destined by the transference situation to love the analyst, the analyst loves the patient inasmuch as he is able to put himself in the patient's place, to identify needs and wishes in the patient and wishes to help her. The analyst is perhaps strangely but rightly detached from this love for the patient, from his identification. This is another analytic paradox: the love of the analyst is only possible because of his detachment (cf. Kristeva, 1983). This detached love will allow the analyst to manage the patient's persecutory anxieties and reactions of hate, a task more relevant to making a psychoanalysis successful than the naïve belief that "love" is the curative force (Friedman, 1998, p. 171). In spite of what some of the authors of the intersubjective school suggest, the relationship between patient and analyst is never the same for both. The intensity of the patient's transference occurs only because of the lack of symmetry in the relationship; this creates a tension in the analytic relationship between asymmetry and mutuality, a tension that needs to be kept, not dissolved (Hoffer, 1996; see also Modell, 1990). Lacan called it "subjective disparity" (Lacan, 1960–61).

Freud believed that the analytic situation itself not only created the possibility for love to occur in transference but, moreover, that love in transference is "provoked by the analytic situation" (1915a, p. 168). The fact that this phenomenon can only be revealed and elucidated in the context of an intimate and peculiar dialogue, where knowledge necessarily passes through an Other, is the radical and privileged uniqueness of psychoanalysis. When psychoanalysts are required to produce evidence, this can only come from the patient's transference, its disruptive presence, its unruly passion, its outrageous persistence, which announces to the world how little our ego is king in its own bedroom, in its own house.

While being unavoidable, love in transference has a very precise and specific reality. This is the stuff of tragedy: the patient lacks the freedom to choose to fall or not to fall in love with the analyst, yet cannot avoid having to take responsibility for her sentiments. The intensity and characteristics (that is, benign or malignant, facilitating or persistently over-eager) of the love developed and experienced in transference will depend to a great extent on the subject's original negotiations at the primary state of helplessness. Emotional failures and psychic breakdowns during this prolonged initial stage of development will create unyielding oral hunger, a yearning for a nurturing mother imago that never truly materialises. Hopefully, these impossible yearnings will be contained by and worked through in the process of analysis. In the context of the treatment, they may be a necessary step towards facilitating the process, allowing the analysis to take place.

Nevertheless, as in the case of Barbara, in many female patients it is most likely and predictable that, sooner or later (as argued earlier in this book), the patient might ask to be loved by the analyst at all costs, at times asking for a mutual pact of negation of reality. If critically severe, this highly eroticised, in contrast to erotic, transference might never relent (Blum, 1973). In the case of Barbara, for example, she was entangled in a malignant predicament in the transference. She appeared to be driven to put herself in masochistic situations, while at the same time desperately trying to run away from them; she could not surrender to the process of the analysis, to give up hope of her "love" being reciprocated by the analyst.

The love of the analyst for the patient is combined but not confused with love for the task, for the work; these facets cannot effectively work without each other. As generous as the analyst's love may be, detachment allows the analyst to understand the absurd aspects of the desire contained in the passionate declarations uttered by the patient. Winnicott spoke of the importance of the "distance between analyst and patient" (1960a, p. 161). Without this distance, the analyst might take the patient's declarations of love as irrefutable proof of his personal qualities and attractiveness.

To be an analyst requires a degree of fervour, of passion for the ideas that the theory of psychoanalysis offers. More than anything else, it is this passion that keeps the analyst alive, real, and good enough for his patients. The analyst will feel genuinely close to the patient whenever the latter allows the former to analyse her – that is, when the insight offered by the analyst is accepted, taken in, and used by the patient for her own benefit, not just to please the analyst. These moments are particularly important when they have been preceded by a period of negativity and malignant resistance in the work of the analysis (Priscilla Roth, private communication, 2003).

Notes

1 This does not exclude the hypothesis of the existence of a primitive identification, the primary narcissism of a pre-object state, as argued in previous chapters.

6

THE QUESTION OF UNCERTAINTY

The demands for (an illusion) of success

In the early 1980s, Michael Rustin described "the social and political affiliations of Kleinian psychoanalysis in Britain" (1991, p. 145). Ten years later, he acknowledged that the historical references had changed radically. Is it possible that first Thatcherism and then Blair's New Labour political ideas have also influenced and changed psychoanalytic *ideals*? (Rustin, 2001). At present, almost two decades later, things seem to have got even worse. Today, listening to contemporary political debates and parliamentary discussions, with speeches full of platitudes, are we perceiving different forms of stupidity and emotional deadness in our political leaders?

In 2001, Rustin referred to the fact that reactionary Thatcherite policies had already started to cause substantial damage to post-war welfare institutions; the socialist and optimistic political hopes of earlier times were faced with the crude realities of an ideology of self-interest, ruthlessness, lack of compassion, materialism, "anomic disintegration, self-seeking, and confusion" (p. 146) that then followed.

Having in Chapter 1 made a plea for the detailed study of single clinical cases as the only valid way of studying psychoanalysis, I would like now to address briefly the question of research in the area of mental health.

In psychoanalytic terms, the ego ideal of individuals evoked by the present political climate, instead of being a guiding ethical point of reference, an inspiring and directing internal agency, has become a destructive, persecuting psychic organisation of control. In trying to prove their own worth (an understandable need), professionals in many areas of society have become alienated by the illusions of the "audit" culture. The pressure is "to produce only good news", thus creating and maintaining an illusion of success (Cooper & Lousada, 2005, p. 61). I suggest that this is the mark of a mutually influential individual and social ideology characterised by a form of symbolic impoverishment (see Kohon, 1999).[1]

In 2005, Andrew Cooper and Julian Lousada described the nature of the contemporary welfare state project: how bureaucratic and useless protocols of regulation, evidence-based practices, distorted outcome studies, phoney targets of research, quality assurance systems, inspection, monitoring, and auditing follow the values of affluent consumerist society and result in the delivery of care that is effectively shallow and driven by fashion. The so-called "free"-market competition has destabilised hospitals and services; it has successfully made the professionals working in them insecure in their positions, leading them to feel doubtful of their knowledge and experience and uncertain about their future. Furthermore, narrow-minded and prejudiced approaches and strategies serve dangerously to avoid "the complexity of ill health, distress, and injustice" (2005, p. 7). Most worryingly, Cooper and Lousada state that

> A central danger of this state of affairs is that propaganda and crude forms of ideological management of reality make their appearance as substitutes for sober engagements with uncomfortable truths. … [Furthermore,] the emergence of forms of discipline, ordering, and surveillance … have a noticeably irrational character … important principles of truth, meaning, and authenticity are in danger of being sacrificed in order to reassure the critical "superintendents" that we are in fact "doing it right" and won't make the same mistakes again.
>
> (2005, pp. 61–62)

The area of mental health is an especially critical example: the emphasis placed on the need for quick results and "efficacy" is often in conflict with the clinicians' assessment of the patients and the appropriate treatment required for each individual (Beck, 1986; Slade & Priebe, 2006). In clinics and hospitals all around the country there does not seem now to be much time for genuine consideration of the personal situation of each patient; again and again, clinicians are urged by institutional managers to conform to protocols and treatment plans that will keep targets on track, avoid potential legal threats, and cast politically motivated statistics in a positive light, citing concern for the safety of patients and others.

In the *Journal of the Balint Society*, Andrew Elder made a comparable point in connection with the work of GPs within the NHS. He described the "clash of cultures" that existed then (2005) between the priorities and attitudes of the Government's policies in Primary Care Trusts[2] and those of Balint-inspired GPs. Some of the characteristics present today in mainstream GP culture include, for example, the by now familiar over-emphasis on apparently "objective" knowledge, clinical parameters set contractually by administrators, so-called "quality" points that attract increasing financial rewards, and 10-minute appointments, all of which undermine continuity of contact between the GPs and their patients.

Elder argued that this represents

> a hefty push back down the always slippery slope towards a more impersonal, disease-centred, and soon-to-be mini-specialist system at primary care level.
>
> (2005, p. 42)

The shift in the politics of health has also considerably affected nursing practices in the NHS, where it is estimated that administrative work occupies as much as 40% of the nurses' weekly tasks.[3] Nurses are supposed to record every so-called "health event"; they are obliged to fill in forms and complete documentation, ensuring that every intervention is recorded and that targets are not only met but accounted for. Similar complaints come from psychologists and psychiatrists working in the NHS, who now spend a large proportion of their time away from clinical work, obliged to satisfy the interminable demands to file information and fill in forms. While the requirement to document events occurring with patients as well as assessments and treatments is a necessary form of accountability, the bureaucratic exaggeration of these processes undermines the clinical expertise of the clinicians involved.

From a psychological point of view, some of the managers and bureaucrats in charge of making fundamental decisions for the general welfare of entire communities appear to suffer from a seriously diminished form of symbolic functioning, dressed up as "rationality", "efficiency", and financial "expediency".[4] Comparable problems are affecting the world of education.[5]

It would be useful to keep clear the difference between the ordinary narcissistic need of a professional who wants to prove his worth and a number of potentially pathological distortions. Scientific researchers can become intoxicated by their own discourse and by what they experience as their scientific achievements. At times, they present the ideology of an ideocratic group of people, in the style of a populist party, hoping that everyone else will follow them. A dialectical movement is thus created: scientific "achievements" are used to gain positions with political power and, in turn, become confused with further scientific achievement; in order to maintain the power, researchers may exaggerate their achievements. The gratification of idealised wishes operates in certain individuals through heroic identifications; for example, some regard themselves as the "saviours" of their discipline, hoping or even claiming that their contribution will rescue their scientific domain from catastrophe and consequent disappearance. It is possible that the heroic vision of sometimes quite limited achievements appears convincing, leading colleagues and admirers to a "blindness of the seeing eye" (Freud, 1895, p. 117) or, as John Steiner has described it, "[turning] a blind eye" to questionable actions (Steiner, 1993).

The excessive expectations of a narcissistic nature that megalomaniac phantasies create hardly disguise the subject's narcissistic vulnerability. If dreams of glorious recognition are not realised, feelings of depression and confusion can emerge, alongside a sense of purposelessness and disillusionment, despair and ineffectiveness. As in other areas of human endeavour, ethical standards and authentic moral values tend to be relaxed at times of crisis for the sake of restoring narcissistic balance.

In response to the demands for simplified results concerning the efficacy of therapeutic psychoanalytic treatment, there is the risk of an equally deficient and mediocre response concerning both the theory and the practice of psychoanalysis. In the last decade or so, there has been a persistent and increasingly intense, often misguided, reactionary shift within certain sectors of psychoanalytic psychotherapy and psychoanalysis; this represented a move towards a highly reductive concept of scientific research that has attempted to constitute itself as an ideal, devaluing the central importance of the single case study. At the same time, the ethical issue of professional accountability in psychoanalysis, important as it is, has been (mis)used to hide institutional conflicts. Accountability has been erroneously confused with measuring the outcomes of therapeutic intervention in ways that neglect the nature of psychoanalysis as such.

The question of uncertainty

The question of the uncertainty of psychoanalytic cure inevitably remains an enormous challenge and a continuing question for those of us who are clinical practitioners. Given the necessary uncertainty at its heart, psychoanalysis is particularly exposed to criticism and psychoanalysts become open to attacks. There are good and searching reasons why research in psychoanalysis is inherently limited; as argued in Chapter 1, there is no model to describe or convey the specificity of the psychoanalytic discipline. Even so, in the present climate, such views as the following can be found:

> Our research efforts obviously need to move both into the comparative study of groups subjected to naturalistic and empirical conditions, as well as to the intense study of individual patients (*N* = 1), based on the direct observation of the psychoanalytic process, as well as *studies where significant aspects of the psychoanalytical process can be evaluated experimentally under different conditions and in alternative clinical designs.*
>
> (Kernberg, 2006; italics added)

By contrast, Thomas Ogden, a year earlier, had written that

> the art of psychoanalysis [is] a process inventing itself as it goes. … Psychoanalysis is a lived emotional experience. As such, it cannot be translated, transcribed, recorded, explained, understood or told in words.
>
> (Ogden, 2005, p. 1)

Ogden's understanding emphasises that the epistemological criteria of validation in psychoanalysis cannot exist outside its own frame of reference, which is highly complicated by the object of enquiry – that of the subject's unconscious and its formations. He sees that the unconscious is an intricate object of study: although it belongs to one particular individual, the influence of the unconscious affects an area between the individual and the social, between self and others, between the inside and the outside, at the very limit of the distinction between the body and the mind. His view is much closer to the reality of psychoanalysis.

How can the psychoanalyst accurately describe the logic of the unconscious, where reasons and causes, pain and pleasure, past and present are inevitably entangled and implicated? Faced with this, Pontalis asked, "Can we do anything but to evoke?" (2000, p. 75; translation modified).

Wilfred R. Bion was more forceful and provocative. In his attempt to study "highly abnormal" personalities, he described the capacity to think in human beings as "rudimentary", arguing that, given this human inadequacy, any field of investigation is essentially limited only "to those phenomena that have the characteristics of the inanimate". Furthermore, he declared that

> We assume that the psychotic limitation is due to an illness: that that of the scientist is not. Investigation of the assumption illuminates disease on the one hand and scientific method on the other. It appears that our rudimentary equipment for "thinking" thoughts is adequate when the problems are associated with the inanimate, but not when the object for investigation is the phenomenon of life itself. *Confronted with the complexities of the human mind the analyst must be circumspect in following even accepted scientific method; its weakness may be closer to the weakness of psychotic thinking than superficial scrutiny would admit.*
>
> (1962b, p. 14; italics added)[6]

To encounter psychoanalysis is inevitably to confront questions: how to account, in psychoanalysis, for the fact that the truth of a subject is not only discovered but also reconstructed or even constructed? How to measure the efficacy of the treatment based on what the patient says, when his speech is the very thing that a psychoanalyst is supposed to question? Parameters used in psychology or in psychiatry are not necessarily relevant nor acceptable in psychoanalysis. Would we be interested in quantifying the "amount of contentment", even were it possible, that a person has achieved through his analysis? Or should we rely on the disappearance of his symptoms? Or perhaps on his life achievements – becoming a banker or a dentist or, for that matter, a psychoanalyst? All such criteria are external and alien to the nature of psychoanalysis – by definition, they paralyse movement and freeze life. How, for example, does the psychoanalyst describe or narrate the unique and intimate relationship where a patient tells a psychoanalyst phantasies, thoughts, and events of his life that he would never dare tell anyone else? How, indeed, can I account for my own responses as an analyst, responses that will have been inspired not only by what I already know, but by what I did not know until I said it, until I happened to utter the words that became my interpretation?

It is difficult for those undertaking research to achieve satisfactory models of explanations. For example, Peter Hobson and Raman Kapur (2005) have studied the belief of psychoanalytic psychotherapists that, not surprisingly, "a principal vehicle for therapeutic change is the analysis of transference between patient and therapist". Most psychoanalytic psychotherapists would agree that this aspect of their technique is what distinguishes their approach from any other therapeutic techniques. The authors of the study thus define the fundamental task for the purpose of doing psychotherapy research as:

> to define what it means to work in the transference, and to study how far psychoanalytic therapists do indeed frame their verbal interpretations so that these take the form of *transference interpretations*.
>
> (Hobson & Kapur, 2005, p. 275)

The authors explored this question in three different ways: they offered an overview of different clinical perspectives on transference interpretations, they studied examples of transference interpretations provided by other researchers, and they reported "an empirical study of the quality, frequency, and distribution of transference interpretations" used (by one of the authors) in the course of psychodynamic assessment interviews in the NHS.

In a paper reporting their conclusions, they stated that:

> one cannot make assumptions about the degree to which different clinicians and different researchers mean the same thing by the term *transference interpretation*. Even when there appears to be much in common among definitions, a closer inspection of the

> quality of interpretations given by different clinicians suggests that wide divergences in technique may be obscured unless explicit examples are given – and even then, much remains to be done to specify the nature of the treatment, as well as the accuracy and appropriateness of interpretations, under study.
>
> (Hobson & Kapur, 2005, p. 289)

This is a well-known fact: different clinicians may give very different definitions and contradictory meanings to the same concept across the whole theoretical body of psychoanalysis – not just to the meaning of "transference interpretation". This state of affairs is, naturally, not conducive to doing psychotherapy research of any sort. Researchers would be attempting to establish agreement on the definition of such a multiplicity of concepts that consensus would be impossible. Towards the end of the article, its two authors declare:

> If it is the case that there are substantial and consistent differences among psychodynamic psychotherapists in their manner of working in the transference ... then it becomes a matter of importance *to devise formal methods to specify and classify such differences*, as a precondition for studying the processes and outcomes of different styles of psychotherapy.
>
> (Hobson & Kapur, 2005, p. 290; italics added)

This is the site of the problem: is it possible, given what is known about the subject of study, "to devise formal methods to specify and classify such differences", as suggested by the authors? Is it possible to develop a privileged method that would secure a true, unambiguous study and certain knowledge of the reality to be investigated? In reporting their study, Hobson and Kapur's final statement is that, "The scientific study of psychotherapy requires both *transparency* and *measurement* of clinical technique" (2005, p. 291; italics added) .

This needs to be put into context: at the last count, there were 500 different forms of psychotherapy in the relevant literature (Karasu, 1986).

Was it not known to Hobson and Kapur, before starting their "empirical study", that psychotherapists and psychoanalysts would not be able to agree on a clear definition and conceptualisation of "transference interpretation"? Did they believe that agreement would be an achievable goal?

Peter Fonagy has also stated the need for methods of "measurement" to identify psychological changes:

> [W]e need *sensitive measurement systems* that identify changes in psychological functioning associated with long-term psychoanalytic psychotherapy that may go beyond symptomatic improvement and indicate benefits that are either valued by clients (or carers) or can be shown to be predictive of relative freedom from future difficulties (prevention).
>
> (2004, p. xxii; italics in the original)

These words come from the "Foreword" to a collection of papers on *Research on Psychoanalytic Psychotherapy with Adults* (Richardson, Kächele & Renlund, 2004). Some of the conclusions put forward by the authors are very interesting. For example, von Wietersheim at al., in their study on the treatment of eating disorders, concluded:

> Direct comparisons between change (successful outcomes) in the field of personality and symptoms show moderate agreement. Symptomatic improvement went along with improvements in the domain of personality; the correlation coefficients ... were only of moderate strength. The question of whether changes in the fields of personality and apparent symptoms coincide or take place in succession, and whether change in one field – e.g. personality – is a requirement for change in another – e.g. symptoms – remains unclear.
>
> (von Wietersheim et al., 2004, p. 12)

They add that

> Successful prediction of improvement in the personality domain could not be achieved. Change in personality could also not be explained by patient variables such as degree of apparent symptoms, duration of illness, number of previous treatments, and so on, or by therapy variables, such as duration and intensity of inpatient therapy.
>
> (2004, p. 12)

Wietersheim et al. concluded that

> parameters affecting the changes shown in inpatients with eating disorders remain unclear.
>
> (2004, p. 13)

Fonagy, commenting on this paper, writes in his "Foreword":

> Perhaps a new approach to *measurement* of individual differences is required by psychoanalytic investigations.
>
> (Fonagy, 2004, p. xxxiii)

In another contribution to this book, Anthony Bateman, in his study of the treatment of borderline personality disorders (BPD), concludes:

> While the results of our study are encouraging, we know neither why patients improve, nor which patients are likely to benefit most from a psychoanalytically orientated treatment. Further development of psychoanalytic approaches to the treatment of BPD will only come about *if we identify the mechanisms of therapeutic change more precisely and decide on the sequencing of interventions and on whom the interventions are to be carried out.*
>
> (Bateman, 2004, p. 131; italics added)

Bateman warns the reader that, if "psychoanalysis is to remain a vibrant and living discipline", then "further research is urgently needed" (2004, p. 132).

More research. More empirical studies. More formal methods. More transparency. More measurements. More sensitivity. And more evidence of effectiveness. It might be worth recalling that, as far as the effectiveness of treatment is concerned, Freud suspected that psychoanalysis could not compete with Lourdes (1933, p. 152).

In an article published in the *World Psychiatry* journal, Fonagy (2015) provides an updated review of outcome studies and meta-analyses of the effectiveness of psychodynamic therapy.

In considering psychodynamic psychotherapy, he writes that

> This review uses a broad definition of psychodynamic treatment as a stance taken to human subjectivity that is inclusive and

> aimed at a comprehensive understanding of the interplay between aspects of the individual's relationship with his/her environment, whether external or internal. It refers to the extraordinary human potential for dynamic self-alteration and self-correction. This definition incorporates a developmental perspective, and assumes limitations on conscious influence, ubiquity of conflict, internal representation of relationships, mental defences, and that complex meanings can be attached to experience.
>
> (Fonagy, 2015, p. 138)

A considerable number of therapies could fit into this very broad definition. The focus of the report is on effectiveness, and Fonagy adopts a "pragmatic" approach; his review uses the researchers' "self-declared allegiance as the guiding principle as to what constitutes PDT (psycho-dynamic therapy)". After reviewing 211 papers, he argues that, surprisingly, different reviews of the same literature appear to reach different conclusions. For example: (a) the conclusions often seemingly reflect the authors' theoretical orientation; (b) the outcomes of individual studies appear to be highly correlated with the first author's affiliation, and (c) the lack of balance and the determination to use statistics primarily for the support of one's own ideas lead to entrenched traditions. The speed of recovery and cost-effectiveness of interventions being the crucial parameter, it would appear that the so-called evidence-based movement in psychotherapy may not have provided a sufficiently meaningful basis for the evidence so strongly desired (Fonagy, 2015).

In the same report, Fonagy also suggested that there is little evidence to indicate that psychodynamic therapy is superior to other therapeutic approaches, arguing that "*Any apparent superiority of long-term psychodynamic therapies is attributable to the prolonged contact between patient and therapist*" (Fonagy, 2015, p. 145; italics added). In other words, the superiority is due to the long-term relationship between patient and therapist and the dynamics of transference and countertransference.

Finally, Fonagy recommends that

> there is considerably more to be achieved by "playful" experimentation, probably driven by advances in bioscience and computational psychiatry.
>
> (Fonagy, 2015, p. 145)

Bioscience designates, collectively, the life sciences; at the same time, it can refer to any one type of science dealing with the structure and behaviour of living things, such as botany, zoology, biochemistry, and anthropology. However, as far as the study of the behaviour of organisms is concerned, such as practiced in ethology and psychology, these disciplines are only covered by the concept of bioscience *as long as there is a clear biological aspect in their application.*

The concept of *computational psychiatry* inhabits an intersectional point between computational neuroscience and psychiatry. These two disciplines both consider and study the potential of new approaches to psychiatric issues; they incorporate methods from other disciplines like neuroscience, behavioural economics, and machine learning (a field of statistics and computer science which gives computer systems the ability to "learn", thus progressively improving performance on a specific task without being explicitly programmed). Computational psychiatry is focused on building mathematical models of neural or cognitive phenomena relevant to psychiatric diseases. The models span a wide range, from biologically detailed models of neurones or networks to abstract models describing high-level cognitive abilities of an organism.

While recognising Fonagy's expertise, it is surely difficult to judge at this point how useful or creative the potential collaboration between these two fields of knowledge might be for the purpose of assessing the outcome of different forms of psychodynamic treatments.

Four months after the above paper was published, Fonagy and colleagues gave an account of a randomised controlled trial to test the effectiveness of long-term psychoanalytic psychotherapy (LTPP) as an alternative to "treatment-as-usual" under UK national guidelines. The research focused on patients with long-standing major depression who had failed at least two different treatments and were considered to have treatment-resistant depression. They were assessed at six-monthly intervals during the 18 months of treatment and at 24, 30, and 42 months' follow-up. The final scores, produced by both observer-based and self-reported depression, showed steeper declines in depression in the group of patients who had undergone psychoanalytic psychotherapy and greater improvements on measures of social adjustment, but

> differences emerged from 24 months post-randomization, with the LTPP group mostly maintaining the gains achieved while

> the control group appeared to be at greater risk of relapse. At 2-year follow-up, almost one-third of the participants receiving LTPP were still in partial remission, compared with only 4% of those in the control group. At that time, 44% of the LTPP group no longer met diagnostic criteria for major depressive disorder, compared with 10% of those receiving [treatment as usual] alone.
>
> (Fonagy et al., 2015, p. 318)

In comparison to other therapeutic interventions, this suggested the usefulness of the psychoanalytic therapeutic approach through *its delayed therapeutic benefit*. Considering the potential implications of such a finding for the inclusion of psychodynamic psychotherapies in the NHS, this may be an important point of reference for future studies.

However, the authors described important limitations of the study:

> First, the design of the study did not allow masking of patients to the treatment allocation, which may have generated an expectation bias. Second, although mixed-effects models are thought to be robust even to selective loss of data, we still failed to collect primary outcome data for over 25% of patients at 42 months, despite an unusually good level of retention for patients with depression of this severity. Third, the differences between the effects associated with the two treatments could have arisen as a result of the disparities between their respective numbers of contact hours, intensity, and quality of case management. Fourth, in spite of robust procedures, randomization yielded a difference between groups in education level, with associated asymmetries in employment and state benefits, which we were forced to adjust for statistically. Reanalysis in which the samples were balanced by selectively excluding patients did not alter the basic pattern of findings. Fifth, while we were concerned to measure outcome over an extended period, we omitted to include an interval depression measure such as the Longitudinal Interval Follow-up Evaluation. Sixth, since the study was planned and conducted by the developers of the intervention, there is a risk of allegiance bias. We tried to minimize this risk by having the primary outcome measure assessments made by

> interviewers who were blinded to the treatment condition. Seventh, these results were delivered by a single provider organization. This may limit generalizability.
>
> (Fonagy et al., 2015, pp. 318–319)

The authors concluded that

> while the benefit of both interventions for this severely affected group of patients with major depressive disorder was limited, *a moderate difference emerged over long-term follow-up in favour of the LTPP condition.* Further studies are needed to replicate this finding, ascertain its clinical utility, understand the mechanisms involved, and identify factors associated with response or non-response to treatment.
>
> (Fonagy et al., 2015, pp. 318–319; italics added)

In general terms, it would appear that the conclusions of psychoanalysts working in the area of research could be summarised thus: (a) there is the need for more precision in the formal methods of research; this would facilitate (b) new approaches and new developments that would enable, in turn, more accurate measurements; (c) there is a prevalent demand for additional transparency and more clearly defined parameters; and (d) there should be more funds and opportunities available to pursue further research.

"Transparency" and "measurement" are taken to be "universal characteristics" of a method of research that would "allow" a given study to be qualified as "scientific"; such accepted characteristics would help to validate its conclusions. Indeed, the authors of psychoanalytic research find it difficult to move away from a certain conventionality in the world of research, thus ignoring the ontological problems presented to them by their object of study.[7] They appear to hope for acceptable explanations and generalisations that would, in turn, create the possibility for predictions, further experiments, and controlled studies. This frame of mind and approach cannot, by definition, sustain singularity and difference. Inevitably, it produces "scientism" in social disciplines like history, anthropology, and psychoanalysis, all of which, necessarily, give special importance to single case studies (see Perelberg, 2005, p. 14). Scientism also creates an illusion of knowing; ironically, it follows the same chimerical path that the omnipotence of the subject's early narcissism never abandons.

Evidence-based medicine

In seeking to establish their own high and acceptable standards, most contemporary models of research take the concept of evidence-based medicine as the most important parameter of reference. But, in modern medicine, the question of evidence is itself not free from controversy. Evidence-based medicine is defined by the idea that what is therapeutic should be decided by a conscious, explicitly rational and sensible use of the best treatment on offer, that this treatment should have been proven effective by scientific research, and that the choice of treatment should accord with criteria of cost-effectiveness, often a controversial issue.

For the last few decades, the internationally recognised *Cochrane Database of Systematic Reviews*, published electronically, has been producing systematic reviews of primary research in human health care and health policy. The reviews follow strict guidelines in order to establish whether or not there is conclusive evidence about a specific treatment; it also covers prevention and rehabilitation. It represents the highest standard in the promotion of evidence-based medicine. This database, together with others, is of enormous and effective help to the health care community.

Nevertheless, in the last few years, several forms of criticism concerning the question of evidence have been appearing in the scientific literature. For example, Kerridge and Saul have argued that

> There is no doubt that the "best available evidence" is an important component of medical decision-making. ... However, [evidence-based medicine] is not an impartial or value-neutral force in modern medicine, and has as much capacity for abuse as any other double-edged sword forged by science.
>
> (2003, p. 314)

These are strong words, still valid today, 15 years after their publication. From a psychological point of view, is it possible that evidence-based medicine can be influenced by the unconscious desire of the people involved in making the decisions?

In a similar vein, Cynthia Mulrow[8] and Kathleen Lohr[9] have earlier argued that

> Judging what constitutes sound evidence can be difficult because of, among other things, the sheer quantity, diversity, and complexity of medical evidence available today; the various scientific methods that have been advanced for assembling, evaluating, and interpreting such information; and the guides for applying medical research evidence to individual patients' situations.
>
> (2001, p. 249)

Reading their article on "Proof and Policy from Medical Research Evidence", which addressed the question of *what* constitutes sound medical research evidence, is a sobering experience. Presented almost two decades ago at a workshop in 2000 on "Evidence: Its Meaning and Uses in Law, Medicine, and Health", they argued that

> Interpreting and judging medical research involves subjective, not solely explicit, processes. Thus, developments in evidence-based medicine are *an aid, not a panacea*, for definitely establishing benefits and harms of medical care.
>
> (2001, p. 249; italics added)

The more data are gathered and compiled, the more difficult it is to compare the patients in the studies with the individual patient actually present in the doctor's surgery. The authors claim that, already in the 1990s, there were 2,000,000 articles on medical research published annually in more than 20,000 biomedical journals; at present, processing this information must be staggering and very difficult. At the same time, the methods used to evaluate such evidence vary, depending entirely upon the questions that are being asked (Mulrow & Lohr, 2001, p. 254). Furthermore, interpreting the results of medical evidence is difficult not only because of the multiplicity of sources, but also because of the variety of research designs (Mulrow & Cook, 1998). Following on from this, it becomes clear that subjective judgement plays a central part in evaluating the different types of evidence. Although finding evidence is absolutely necessary and its importance cannot be minimised, it is not as "objective" a process as we are led to believe.

In the present political climate it is easy to forget that the researchers who first spoke of "evidence-based medicine" wanted to emphasise *the probabilistic aspects of medical care* (Sackett & Guyau, 1992). Making decisions regarding the health care of individuals is an activity based on a multiplicity of sources of information gathered in the context of large groups and populations. Thus, they advocate a *quantitative* approach to medical practice. Aimed at replacing mere "opinion" and the individual clinician's experience, they appeal to statistical associations and differences. In other words, they demand numerical results, which can then be turned into scientific and objective proof.

Nevertheless, the comparison between sample groups provides little information, if any, regarding the responses of the individual to a given treatment. The information obtained from the study of large groups might not indicate the proportion of individuals who have improved or recovered as a result of treatment. Statistical comparisons between groups do not directly address the clinical significance of the medical intervention. Commenting on this aspect of the practice of evidence-based medicine, Mulrow and Lohr state that

> accurate precision or proof of causality (or both) applicable to real-life settings is difficult and relies on judgement regarding the magnitude of probability and uncertainty (reasonable doubt) that one considers as acceptable proof.
>
> (2001, p. 258)

Antonio Damasio has pointedly explained that "conscious and rational" decisions are not easily available to people. Decisions made on the principle of rational consideration of all factors present in any human circumstance would take an unacceptably long time; the human mind could not take into account the range of all possible ramifications. To take all possible rational options into consideration before making a decision, "get a lot of paper and a pencil sharpener, and a large desk, and do not expect anybody to wait until you are finished" (Damasio, 1994, p. 172). Quoting the work of Amos Tversky and Daniel Kahneman (1973), who demonstrated that the objective reasoning we believe we employ in common decisions is far less effective and helpful than it seems and ought to be, Damasio argues that

> even if our reasoning strategies were perfectly tuned, it appears they would not cope well with the uncertainty and complexity of personal and social problems. The fragile instruments of rationality need special assistance.
>
> (1994, p. 191)

Damasio, a professor of neurology, comes close to a psychoanalytic view when he asserts that his concept of rationality necessarily includes the personal desires, unconscious drives, and biological instincts of the subject. Inevitably, this makes the picture concerning rational decisions "even more complicated" (see 1994, pp. 165–201).

Another medical author, M. R. Tonelli[10] (2001), has taken the criticism of evidence-based medicine further and states that

> the type of knowledge gained from clinical research, referred to ... as "empirical evidence", is itself insufficient. ... A gap exists between empirical evidence and clinical practice. Proponents of evidence-based medicine have clearly acknowledged one aspect of this gap: the part that requires the consideration of values, both patient and professional, prior to arriving at medical decisions. Not as clearly recognised, however, is the gap that exists due to the fact that empirical evidence is not directly applicable to individual patients, as the knowledge gained from clinical research does not directly answer the primary clinical question of what is best for the patient at hand.
>
> (2001, p. 1435)

Tonelli specifically argues that proponents of evidence-based medicine do not take into account the value of *clinical experience* in the process of making their judgements.

In justifying the achievements of evidence-based medicine in relation to cost-effectiveness, the actual results are not as encouraging as might be expected. The past decades have shown that the individual doctor in clinical practice deviates considerably from research-based recommendations (Eddy, 1996). Moreover, it is acknowledged that there is wide variation in how cost-effectiveness is defined and applied (Havighurst, Hutt, McNeil & Miller, 2001; Jacobson, 2001) For example, the simplest way of applying the criteria of cost-effectiveness is to compare two interventions aimed at the same outcome. But, even at this simple level, the analysis of cost-effectiveness is laden with methodological difficulties and subjective value judgements (Havighurst, Hutt, McNeil & Miller, 2001).

Finally, a paper published in the *Australian and New Zealand Journal of Surgery* (Little, 2003) suggests that, concerning modern evidence-based medicine, there are different features that need further exploration and discussion. Some of them are: (a) its reductionism, seeking to "reduce the basis of explanation to something simpler and more fundamental"; (b) its privileging of restricted kinds of evidence, treating qualitative research with contempt, as if it were *not science*; as a consequence of this prejudice, researchers feel the pressure to create instruments of research that, cast in the scientific mould, "can work only with qualities that are already known and defined"; (c) its dependence on the application of randomised controlled trials (considered to be the "gold-standard"), whereas these trials pose serious ethical and significant strategic problems; (d) its capacity to eliminate individuals in favour of categories, promoting uniformity of treatment not always suitable to the individual patient, etc.

Although Little described his paper as a "gentle" critique of evidence-based medicine, his criticisms are not insignificant. He claims that

> What is taught in medical school … privileges numerical and scientific evidence, to the exclusion of the subjective and qualitative evidence. And yet, *it is in the subjective, symptomatic and qualitative aspects of human existence that the health endeavour finds its justification.*
>
> (2003, p. 178; italics added)

In the same issue of *World Psychiatry* mentioned above (October 2015), Dan J. Stein,[11] in his "Editorial", refers to Khan and Brown's work (Stein, 2015), which emphasised the fact that, in contrast to early investigations, in recent antidepressant trials the drug–placebo differences had been smaller. Stein, in describing how mental disorders such as depression cannot easily be defined, argues that a considerable number of causal mechanisms are likely to be involved in the pathogenesis and treatment of mental disorders, including depression. Further, quoting authors like Klein and Ross (1993) and Fountoulakis and Moller (2011), Stein declares that

> The reliance of modern clinical research on randomized placebo-controlled trials has led to an ever growing data-base demonstrating that *placebo is a remarkably powerful intervention for a range of psychiatric and medical conditions, including milder cases of depression.*
>
> (Stein, 2015, p. 258; italics added)

The placebo effect is of fundamental importance for the understanding and development of all projects concerning evidence-based medicine. Benedetti, after performing a standard double-blind randomised controlled trial on a painkiller, demonstrated that the administered drug performed better than the placebo. Nevertheless, when he gave the same drug to another group of volunteers without telling them what he was giving them, the drug did not produce any effect: it was completely ineffective for the relief of pain. That the placebo effect alone can relieve pain has long been known, but Benedetti's work shows how the actual administration of a drug can activate an unknown and complex sequence of biochemical reactions in a subject's brain (Benedetti et al., 2003; see also Colloca et al., 2008).

Newer research is studying the biochemical/neurological processes in the brain relating to placebo – as illustrated in the *Horizon* programme recently shown, *The Placebo Experiment: Can My Brain Cure My Body?* (BBC2, 11 October 2018). The belief in the placebo treatment appeared to trigger, in about half of people, the release of neurochemicals within the body that are analgesic. It is possible now to consider that well-designed trials and studies would support, not negate, the importance of context and clinical encounter. In the *Horizon* documentary, Dr Michael Mosley, the programme's director, made the important point that those patients who received a longer (30-minute rather than 10-minute) consultation with the doctors were more likely to benefit from the placebo treatment.

Miller and Kaptchuk (2008) have argued that the term "placebo" should be replaced by "contextual healing": in their opinion, this would describe much more accurately the process and effect of healing, understood as the result of the context of the clinical encounter rather than the specific medicine and/or treatment given.

The clinical encounter: this is where we have arrived, in the end – a matter of transference and countertransference. This may yet be the most important factor in the effectiveness of a treatment.

Notes

1 In symbolic impoverishment, the subject finds it difficult to experience sympathy for the other's suffering; in the worst of cases, the subject may not find any meaning in sentiments of generosity or

compassion. Concepts, ideas, fantasies, tentative impressions, hypotheses, make-believe, and speculative thoughts can only be understood in terms of concrete actions; imagination is limited, frequently accompanied by unconvincing rationalisations. Subjects remain observers, not active participants; responsibility for the subject's behaviour, or for its consequences, lies outside the self.

2 Primary Care Trusts (PCTs) were part of the NHS in England from 2001 to 2013. They were largely administrative bodies, responsible for commissioning primary, community, and secondary health services from providers, spending around 80% of the total NHS budget. PCTs were abolished on 31 March 2013, their work taken over by Clinical Commissioning Groups (CCGs). At present, there is a similar, or even worse, feeling of discontent with the work of the CCGs. The NHS was established in the UK in 1948. The founding principles were that services should be comprehensive, universal, and free at the point of delivery for people ordinarily resident in the UK.

3 *Patients Not Paperwork – Bureaucracy Affecting Nurses in the NHS* (Cunningham, Kennedy, Nwolisa, Callard & Wike, 2012) was an important report by the NHS Institute for Innovation and Improvement describing the position of the nursing staff in the NHS. The Institute, which closed in March 2013, was a special health authority of the NHS in England, helping the NHS to transform healthcare for patients and the public. *Organising Care at the NHS Front Line – Who Is Responsible?* (Ham & Berwick, 2017), written from a medical doctors' point of view and published by The King's Fund (an independent charity working to improve health and care in England), offers passing but interesting comments concerning the work of the nurses in the NHS. Significantly, it was reported by *Nursing Times* (Somerville & Morrison, 2018) that two senior charge nurses at NHS Ayrshire and Arran won a case for recruiting an administrative assistant, freeing up their time and consequently allowing them to be more visible and active as clinical leaders.

4 To understand the effect of managers in the health and educational professions, see Andrè Spicer's *Business Bullshit* (2018).

5 In *The Very Thought of Education: Psychoanalysis and the Impossible Professions* (2009), Deborah P. Britzman suggests that one aspect of the problems faced by education may be that, "If only seen as a technical skill, the language of teaching suffers from what Gregorio Kohon (2007) calls 'symbolic impoverishment'."

6 I am grateful to Sebastián J. Kohon for drawing my attention to this quotation of Bion (personal communication, 2010).

7 A great majority of researchers would perhaps agree with Peter Fonagy, who declared that "Our aim should be to assist the movement

of psychoanalysis toward *science* ". Nevertheless, I would suspect that not all psychoanalysts would necessarily want to "ensure a future for psychoanalysis and psychoanalytic therapies *within psychiatry*" (Fonagy, 2003, p. 73, 80; italics added).

8 Cynthia Mulrow is the Senior Deputy Editor of the academic journal, *Annals of Internal Medicine*, and an adjunct Clinical Professor of Medicine at the University of Texas Health Science Center at San Antonio. Past positions that she has held include: Director of the San Antonio Cochrane Collaboration Center (1994–2000) and the San Antonio Evidence-based Practice Center (1997–2000). She was elected to the American Society for Clinical Investigation in 1997, honoured as a Master of the American College of Physicians in 2005, and elected to the Institute of Medicine in 2008.

9 Kathleen N. Lohr is a Distinguished Fellow in Health Services Research, RTI International. She was the founding director of the Research Triangle Institute, University of North Carolina (Evidence-based Practice Center, as of 2007, where she is now a senior advisor). In 2005, she was awarded the Avedis Donabedian Outcomes Research Lifetime Achievement Award by the International Society of Pharmacoeconomics & Outcomes Research. In 2007, RTI honoured her with the Margaret Elliott Knox Excellence Award.

10 Professor, Division of Pulmonary and Critical Care Medicine; Section Head, University of Washington Medical Center; Training Director, Pulmonary and Critical Care Medicine Fellowship.

11 Department of Psychiatry and Mental Health, and Director, MRC Unit on Anxiety and Stress Disorders, Groote Schuur Hospital, both at the University of Cape Town.

7

WHAT IS TO BE DONE?

In *Madness of the Day*, Maurice Blanchot wrote,

> I had been asked: Tell us "just exactly" what happened. A story? I began: I am not learned; I am not ignorant. I have known joys. That is saying too little. I told them the whole story and they listened, it seems to me, with interest, at least in the beginning. But the end was a surprise to all of us. "That was the beginning", they said. "Now get down to the facts."
>
> (Blanchot, 1973, p. 18)

Upon reading Blanchot's text, we discover that the demand for the subject to tell the story comes from an eye doctor and a psychiatrist, both representing the order imposed by an established authoritarian world: the demand for a story to be told has inevitably turned into an interrogation. Commenting on Blanchot's text, Levinas (1975) described how it was impossible for a subject to tell the whole story – even if he tried to. The reader is left with the feeling that something is left out, something that is beyond a logical but repressive world. That "something" is not easily comprehensible in our relationships with others: it belongs to the madness of the day (the title of the story).

This short narrative forces the reader to wish for the clear understanding that is missing from the text. While the reader feels compelled to give a meaning to it, the narrator himself admits to having lost the sense of it. A story can be demanded, but this does not necessarily mean that it can be told. A version of a past might be offered, but this does not suggest that it can be reconstructed.

There is no beginning or ending, there will be no outcome, no final conclusion to be drawn.

Patients in analysis are also expected to tell the analyst their story. Here, inevitably, something will always be left out. The analyst is supposed to listen to the story without attempting an interrogation. Outside, in the world beyond the consulting room, psychoanalysts face the demand to tell their own story. The command is: "Get down to the facts, tell us 'just exactly' what happens, give us the evidence."

What can we say? The "reasonable" insistence that psychoanalysts should be able to construct generalisations about their discipline is, in fact, incongruous and inappropriate. At the same time, there is often a wish to provide the evidence demanded – a wish that, although understandable, is misplaced.

Do psychoanalysts have a story to tell? The answer requires immersing ourselves in both our theoretical and our clinical praxes, constantly moving between the precision of poetry and the intuition of science (Nabokov, 1948). Psychoanalysts are interested in what constitutes the elements that make a person or an event distinct. As Isaiah Berlin said of historians, psychoanalysts too are concerned to paint "a portrait which conveys the unique pattern of experience" (1996, p. 22). How do we arrive at our conclusions? Is it possible to develop a science of a single object, of one particular subject? The authorities want protocols, and, inevitably, to prove one's worth has always been a true dilemma for the psychoanalyst; even so, the question should not and cannot be dismissed. In the meantime, we witness how "the best minds of my generation" (Ginsberg, 1956, p. 126) drag themselves through the cul-de-sac of scientism in an environment that is sinking in the bureaucratic mire.

Psychoanalysis works through abductive inference. Hypotheses are held awaiting further confirmation; they are put forward as questions.[1] In contrast to an inductive inference, abduction is the process of forming explanatory hypotheses. During this process, many hypotheses are put forward to explain a fact – but only a few would be viewed as satisfactory. That an explanation might make meaningful sense does not suggest that there is only the one explanation, nor even that it would be the best one. Abduction allows us to infer *a* as an explanation of *b*: the precondition *a* may be abduced from the consequence *b*. There might be many possible explanations for any process that we observe, but we tend to abduce a single explanation, which represents a form of reasoning through successive approximation. Under this principle, an explanation is valid if it is the best possible explanation for a set of known data. For Peirce, abduction is the only logical operation that is capable of introducing new ideas (1903, p. 171; see also Eisele, 1985; Fabbrichesi & Marietti, 2006).

Being a subjective discipline, objectivity in psychoanalysis is neither attainable nor desirable; although there is a potential for a multiplicity of interpretations, there is only one experience, "that ... which the analyst ... had with his patient" (Bion, 1994, p. 7). It is up to the individual psychoanalyst to legitimise that experience. Not all patients are the same: for each psychoanalyst, the challenge is to understand and apply subtle modifications and discriminating and perspicacious adaptations to each individual patient, bearing in mind the state of mind of the patient at a given moment in the transference. The analyst's usual form of an interpretation, "I wonder if ", "it sounds as if", is not a definite conclusion that then becomes a general law. And yet, psychoanalysis appears to be the only systematic way of understanding the human mind in all its living complexity. For this very reason, the best-suited "instrument of research" for the study of the human mind may be another human mind (Dermen, 2001).

Psychoanalytic knowledge is not linear; it is always partial, forever changing in a dynamic and dialectical movement. James Rose and Graham Shulman have recently described the mind itself as a non-linear, complex system, where predictions of any given response to any one stimulus are difficult, if not impossible. For these authors, a central notion in the study of complex systems is "the strange factor" (described originally by David Ruelle, 1980). As defined by Rose,

> It refers to a pattern of cyclical dynamic motion towards which such a system tends when responding to external stimuli, which disturb its internally determined process in some way. ... In psychoanalysis, it can be applied in understanding the patterns of internal representations and internal object relationships, or patterns of affect that can be observed in the transference and countertransference interaction.
>
> (Rose & Shulman, 2016, p. 7)

It conveys not only the absence of a unique, unidimensional meaning, but also the need to place each formation in its context, allowing for diverse – although not infinite – levels of interpretation. It accounts for the symbolic significance of a past conflict as well as for the symbolism of the conflict in the present. Additionally, the application of the ideas of chaos theory to the understanding of therapeutic action is discussed in a number of papers (Rose & Shulman, 2016). Perhaps over-optimistically, they end the book by saying, "Taking the mind to be a non-linear system opens new avenues of research which can be supported by newly emerging statistical methods" (p. 186).

In psychoanalysis, there is no unified narrative that would bring together all theoretical developments and clinical facts. It is a subjective discipline defined by the need to reflect upon one's own self and behaviour. There can be no end to this self-reflection, for psychoanalysis is created and sustained by it. This accounts for the endless diverse readings that Freud's texts offer, as well as the multiplicity of theories that exist within the psychoanalytic field. As a discipline, psychoanalysis survives thanks to its persistence in the self-reflection rooted in its very existence.

Eric Santner, in his book *On the Psychotheology of Everyday Life* (2001), introduced a distinction between the global and the universal, which is worth considering here. In the global view, every stranger is ultimately familiar; one understands his strangeness as a function of a different vocabulary – in other words, if I could only understand the other's language, I would then be able to understand him. The assumption is that words, ideas, and/or culture can be translated from one language to another; there is no challenge in facing the unfamiliar. The strange and unfamiliar of the other are made "known" through a reference to one's own universe, to one's own language, to one's own theory. In the universal view, the interpretation of the unknown is structured around a necessary openness to the strangeness of the other, the very locus of universality. The possibility of commonality, Santner argues, is given by the fact that every familiar is strange, unique, and singular. Moreover, the objects of study (as well as the subject doing the study) are strangers to themselves for the very reason that they each have an unconscious. In this way of understanding, the Oedipus complex makes real sense (that is, becomes universal) when it is (re)-discovered in a specific moment of a clinical session; otherwise, it is devoid of meaning. The global might appear in our theory, but it is the universal (of the singular case) that defines the specificity of psychoanalysis. Santner gives an example taken from Žižek (1997): we truly come to understand (the global aspect of) a language when we begin to know the (universal) meaning of those words that are not translatable – that is, when we perceive the failures of translation.[2]

Intrinsically, psychoanalysis, anthropology, history, and other social sciences share a similar stance: they study the singular being (in the consulting room), the particular culture (in the jungle, mountain, island, etc.), or significant events of the past. They arrive at universal conclusions only through being open to the strangeness of each individual object of study. To compare them to other disciplines, with different objects, dissimilar methods, and opposed aims would not only be unfair, but also mystifying. Elizabeth Spillius (2003) argued that, in psychoanalysis, it would be futile to promote a type of research based not on the universal but on the global, borrowed from other types of knowledge: psychiatry, developmental psychology, infant research, attachment theory, and so forth. Of course, this does not mean that psychoanalysis should ignore the discoveries of other disciplines. Sira Dermen (2001) has convincingly expressed her scepticism of the cross-disciplinary fertilisation of psychoanalysis with "related" sciences (that is, the biological sciences). Similarly, Michael Feldman (2001) has argued against the seduction of the apparent certainty and respectability offered by methods of investigation other than specifically psychoanalytic ones.

Through the work of Husserl, we came to understand that knowledge of the world is achieved through and by human subjectivity. Later, through the work of Freud, Althusser, and Foucault, we learned that the knowing subject is subjectified – in other words, subjected to (and subjugated by) social and historical contingencies as much as by his own unconscious and ideology. Therefore, it is questionable that the analyst should be there to "teach" the patient the meaning of his actions. The analyst is not there medically to "cure" the patient and certainly not to indoctrinate nor save him. Instead, through listening, the analyst tries not to interfere with the process of learning from the other.

J.-B. Pontalis wrote:

> Humility in the presence of the unconscious. … Let's not be in a hurry to translate. … Let's agree to be exposed to this passion, to this rage, to this wailing, to these silences, to all forms of this *excess*, in full ignorance of what incited it. Allow ourselves to be touched, wounded and demolished in our own *being*. Keep company with the shadows so that we may dream, if possible, in

> this darkness interrupted by flashes of light, in order to approach what is radically other, what the other feels as being foreign but from which they cannot escape.
>
> J.-B. Pontalis (2000, pp. 10–11; italics in original)

The specific feature of psychoanalysis, which makes it unlike any other discipline, is that the encounter between a patient and an analyst falls within the limits of an ethics of alterity – the recognition and acceptance that the other person is different. This aspect of the encounter has been significantly illuminated by the work of Levinas. In his view, alterity appears as a non-reciprocal relationship, sometimes surprising, often unpredictable:

> The Other as Other is not only an alter ego: the Other is what I myself am not. The Other is this, not because of the Other's character, or physiognomy, or psychology, but because of the Other's very alterity.
>
> (Levinas, 1987, p. 84)

The patient's speech becomes meaningful through the analyst's listening, which changes the narrative offered by the patient. Nevertheless, it is not the analyst who creates the meaning of the dream, the slip of the tongue, or the symptom for the patient. The unconscious meaning unfolds through the discourse of the patient, revealed, as it were, in the words of the analyst by the analyst's capacity to listen. Furthermore, the practice of psychoanalytic listening resists codification; its technique cannot be prescribed, nor can it be restricted to the contents offered by a manual of therapeutic intervention. The clinical encounter is not limited by epistemological certainties. The challenging ethical question still facing the clinician today is, how do I learn from the patient? This is at the core of the epistemology of psychoanalysis (Casement, 1985), an epistemology that pays special respect to the "complications, subtleties, and variations of human relationships, evident on the patient's side as much as on the analyst's" (Kohon, 1986, p. 72; see also, 2018).

Evidence cannot be given. Proof cannot be provided. Carlo Ginzburg argues that psycho-analysis is a form of conjectural knowledge, an indirect, presumptive, intuitive knowledge based on the study of individual cases. Ginzburg, with undisguised admiration and defiance, brings together psychoanalysis with the science of the physician and the historian, all highly qualitative disciplines. As argued by him, psychoanalysis is a discipline based on details outside conscious control: "infinitesimal traces permit the comprehension of a deeper, otherwise unattainable reality: traces – more precisely, symptoms (in the case of Freud), clues (in the case of Sherlock Holmes)" (Ginzburg, 1989, p. 101).

In the end, as psychoanalysts, we cannot simplify what is extraordinarily multi-layered and exceptionally complex. Psychoanalysis does not aim to reach a position where its theory and practice will be able to give a full and final account of its subject.

Not now.

Not in the future.

Notes

1 The term "abduction" was coined by Charles Sanders Peirce (1903), the American philosopher, mathematician, and scientist, in his work on the logic of science. He introduced it to denote a type of non-deductive inference, different from the already familiar inductive type.

2 Santner's book is based on a study of the Jewish philosopher Franz Rosenzweig and his relationship to Freud.

REFERENCES

Alford, C. F. (1992). *The Psychoanalytic Theory of Greek Tragedy*. New Haven, CT: Yale University Press.

Anderson, R. (2017). Discussion of the case of Bento. *International Journal of Psychoanalysis, 98* (5): 1433–1441.

Aulagnier, P. (1975). *The Violence of Interpretation: From Pictogram to Statement*. Hove: Brunner-Routledge, 2001.

Balibar, E. (1994). Subjection and subjectivation. In J. Copjec (Ed.), *Supposing the Subject*. New York: Verso.

Bateman, A. W. (2004). Psychoanalytically oriented day-hospital treatment for borderline personality disorder: Theory, problems, and practice. In P. Richardson, H. Kächele, & C. Renlund (Eds.), *Research on Psychoanalytic Psychotherapy with Adults*. London: Karnac.

Beck, U. (1986). *The Risk Society*. London: Sage.

Benedetti, F., Maggi, G., Lopiano, L., Lanotte, M., Rainero, I., Vighetti, S., et al. (2003). Open versus hidden medical treatments: The patient's knowledge about a therapy affects the therapy outcome. *Prevention & Treatment, 6* (No. 1, June).

Benjamin, J. (1988). The alienation of desire: Women's masochism and ideal love. In J. L. Alpert (Ed.), *Psychoanalysis and Women: Contemporary Reappraisals*. Hillsdale, NJ: Analytic Press.

Bergeret, J. (1974). The child of the night. *Revue Française de Psychanalyse, 38*: 969–984.

Berlin, I. (1996). *The Sense of Reality: Studies in Ideas and Their History*. London: Pimlico.

Bernstein, D. (1983). The female superego: A different perspective. *International Journal of Psychoanalysis, 64*: 187–201.

Berto, F. (2009). *There's Something about Gödel: The Complete Guide to the Incompleteness Theorem*. Chichester: Wiley-Blackwell.

Bion, W. R. (1957). Differentiation of the psychotic from the non-psychotic personalities. In *Second Thoughts*. London: Heinemann, 1967.

Bion, W. R. (1959). Attacks on linking. In *Second Thoughts*. London: Heinemann, 1967.
Bion, W. R. (1962a). The psycho-analytic study of thinking. *International Journal of Psychoanalysis, 43*: 306–310, Reprinted in *Second Thoughts*. London: Heinemann, 1967.
Bion, W. R. (1962b). *Learning from Experience*. London: Heinemann.
Bion, W. R. (1963). *Elements of Psycho-Analysis*. London: Heinemann.
Bion, W. R. (1965). *Transformations: Change from Learning to Growth*. London: Tavistock.
Bion, W. R. (1970). *Attention and Interpretation: A Scientific Approach to Insight in Psycho-Analysis and Groups*. London: Tavistock.
Bion, W. R. (1994). *Clinical Seminars and Other Works*, ed. F. Bion. London: Karnac.
Blanchot, M. (1973). *The Madness of the Day*, trans. L. Davis. York: Station Hill Press, 1981.
Bleger, J. (1967). Psycho-analysis of the psycho-analytic frame. *International Journal of Psychoanalysis, 48*: 511–519. Reprinted in *Symbiosis y Ambigüedad*. Buenos Aires: Paidós. [*Symbiosis and Ambiguity: A Psychoanalytic Study*, trans. L. Bleger & J. Churcher. London: Routledge/The Institute of Psychoanalysis, 2013].
Bloom, H. (1986). Freud, the greatest modern writer [Book review]. *New York Times*, 23 March, p. 26.
Blum, H. (1973). The concept of erotized transference. *Journal of the American Psychoanalytic Association, 21*: 61–76.
Britton, R. (2003). *Sex, Death and the Superego: Experiences in Psychoanalysis*. London: Karnac.
Britzman, D. P. (2009). *The Very Thought of Education: Psychoanalysis and the Impossible Professions*. Albany, NY: State University of New York Press.
Bronstein, C. (2014). On the excess of nothing: Discussion of J.-B. Pontalis, "No, Twice No". *International Journal of Psychoanalysis, 95* (3): 563–571.
Browne, H., & Streeruwitz, A. (2017). Foreword: Reflections on the greening of psychoanalysis conference. In R. J. Perelberg & G. Kohon (Eds.), *The Greening of Psychoanalysis: André Green's New Paradigm in Contemporary Theory and Practice*. London: Karnac.
Bruner, J. (1990). *Acts of Meaning*. Cambridge, MA: Harvard University Press.
Byatt, A. S. (1985). *Still Life*. New York: Macmillan.
Caldwell, L. (1995). An interview with André Green. *New Formations, 26*: 15–35.
Casement, P. (1985). *On Learning from the Patient*. London: Tavistock.
Castoriadis, C. (1987). *The Imaginary Institution of Society*. Cambridge: Polity Press.

Castoriadis, C. (1988). Logique, imagination, reflexion [Lecture presented to the colloquium on The Unconscious and Science, University of Paris-X (Nanterre), 5–6 March]. In R. Dorey (Ed.), *L'Inconscient et la science*. Paris: Dunod, 1991. [Logic, imagination, reflection, trans. D. A. Curtis. *American Imago, 49* (1992): 3–33.]

Castoriadis, C. (1997). Psychoanalysis and politics. In *World in Fragments: Writings on Politics, Society, Psychoanalysis, and the Imagination*. Stanford, CA: Stanford University Press.

Chasseguet-Smirgel, J. (1964). Feminine guilt and the Oedipus complex. In J. Chasseguet-Smirgel (Ed.), *Female Sexuality*. London: Karnac, 1985.

Chasseguet-Smirgel, J. (1995). "Creative writers and day-dreaming": A commentary. In E. S. Person, P. Fonagy, & S. A. Figueira (Eds.), *On Freud's "Creative Writers and Day-Dreaming"*. New Haven, CT: Yale University Press.

Chodorow, N. (1978). *The Reproduction of Mothering: Psychoanalysis and the Reproduction of Gender*. Berkeley, CA: University of California Press.

Cohen, T. (1999). *Jokes: Philosophical Thought on Joking Matters*. Chicago, IL: University of Chicago Press.

Colloca, L., Tinazzi, M., Recchia, S., Le Pera, D., Fiaschi, A., Benedetti, F., et al. (2008). Learning potentiates neurophysiological and behavioural placebo analgesic responses. *Pain, 139*: 306–314.

Coltart, N. (1987). Diagnosis and assessment for suitability for psychoanalytic psychotherapy. *British Journal of Psychotherapy, 4* (2). Reprinted in *Slouching Towards Bethlehem ... And Further Psychoanalytic Explorations*. London: Free Association Books, 1992.

Coltart, N. (1988). The assessment of psychological-mindedness in the diagnostic interview. *British Journal of Psychiatry, 153*: 819–820.

Cooper, A., & Lousada, J. (2005). *Borderline Welfare: Feeling and Fear of Feeling in Modern Welfare*. London: Karnac.

Crick, P. (2014). Selecting a patient or initiating a psychoanalytic process? *International Journal of Psychoanalysis, 95* (3): 465–484.

Cunningham, L., Kennedy, J., Nwolisa, F., Callard, L., & Wike, C. (2012). *Patients Not Paperwork – Bureaucracy Affecting Nurses in the NHS*. London: NHS Institute for Innovation and Improvement. Available at: www.qualitasconsortium.com/index.cfm/reference-material/fundamentals/patients-not-paperwork

Damasio, A. R. (1994). *Descartes' Error: Emotion, Reason and the Human Brain*. London: Papermac, 1996.

Dermen, S. (2001). What do psychoanalysts know about the mind and what is its evidential basis? *Bulletin of the British Psycho-Analytical Society, 37*: 6.

Deutsch, H. (1932). On female homosexuality. In R. Fliess (Ed.), *The Psychoanalytic Reader* (pp. 195–207). New York: International Universities Press, 1948.

Deutsch, H. (1944). *Female Psychology, Vols. 1 & 2.* New York: Grune & Stratton.
Eddy, D. M. (1996). Benefit language criteria that will improve quality while reducing costs. *Journal of the American Medical Association, 275*: 650–657.
Eigen, M. (1999). *Toxic Nourishment.* London: Karnac.
Eisele, C. (Ed.) (1985). Peirce, the scientist. In *Historical Perspectives on Peirce's Logic of Science: A History of Science.* Amsterdam: Mouton.
Elder, A. (2005). Balint and the clash of cultures [Keynote Address, Oxford 2004]. *Journal of the Balint Society, 33.*
Ey, H., Bernard, P. & Brisset, C. (1965). *Manuel de psychiatrie.* Paris: Masson et Cie.
Fabbrichesi, R., & Marietti, S. (2006). *Semiotics and Philosophy in Charles Sanders Peirce.* Newcastle-upon-Tyne: Cambridge Scholars Publishing, 2008.
Faimberg, H. (2005). *The Telescoping of Generations: Listening to the Narcissistic Links between Generations.* London: Routledge.
Fast, I. (1984). *Gender Identity.* Hillsdale, NJ: Analytic Press.
Feldman, M. (2001). What do psychoanalysts know about the mind? What is the evidential basis for this knowledge? *Bulletin of the British Psycho-Analytical Society, 37*: 4.
Fliegel, Z. O. (1973). Feminine psychosexual development in Freudian theory: A historical reconstruction. *Psychoanalytic Quarterly, 42*: 385–408.
Fliegel, Z. O. (1986). Women's development in analytic theory: Six decades of controversy. In J. L. Alpert (Ed.), *Psychoanalysis and Women: Contemporary Reappraisals.* Hillsdale, NJ: Analytic Press.
Fonagy, P. (2003). Psychoanalysis today. *World Psychiatry, 2* (2): 73–80.
Fonagy, P. (2004). Foreword. In P. Richardson, H. Kächele, & C. Renlund (Eds.), *Research on Psychoanalytic Psychotherapy with Adults.* London: Karnac.
Fonagy, P. (2015). The effectiveness of psychodynamic psychotherapies: An update. *World Psychiatry, 14* (2): 137–150.
Fonagy, P., Rost, F., Carlyle, J., McPherson, S., Thomas, R., Pasco Fearon, R. M., et al. (2015). Pragmatic randomized controlled trial of long-term psychoanalytic psychotherapy for treatment-resistant depression: The Tavistock Adult Depression Study (TADS). Research report. *World Psychiatry, 14* (3): 312–321.
Forrester, J. (2017a). If *p*, then what? Thinking in cases. In *Thinking in Cases* (pp. 1–24). Cambridge: Polity Press.
Forrester, J. (2017b). On Kuhn's case: Psychoanalysis and the paradigm. In *Thinking in Cases* (pp. 25–64). Cambridge: Polity Press.
Forrester, J. (2017c). The psychoanalytic case: Voyeurism, ethics and epistemology in Robert Stoller's *Sexual Excitement.* In *Thinking in Cases* (pp. 65–88). Cambridge: Polity Press.

Fountoulakis, K. N., & Moller, H. J. (2011). Efficacy of antidepressants: A re-analysis and re-interpretation of the Kirsch data. *International Journal of Neuropsychopharmacology, 14*: 405–412.
Freud, S. (1893). Case Histories: Fräulein Elisabeth von R. *Studies on Hysteria. S.E. 2.*
Freud, S. (1895). (with Breuer, J.). *Studies on Hysteria. S.E. 2.*
Freud, S. (1899). Screen memories. *S.E. 3.*
Freud, S. (1900). Letter from Sigmund Freud to Wilhelm Fliess, 1 February. In *The Complete Letters of Sigmund Freud to Wilhelm Fliess 1887–1904*, trans. and ed. J. M. Masson. Cambridge, MA: Harvard University Press, 1985.
Freud, S. (1905). On psychotherapy. *S.E. 7.*
Freud, S. (1906). Letter from Sigmund Freud to C. G. Jung, 6 December. In W. McGuire (Ed.), *The Freud/Jung Letters: The Correspondence Between Sigmund Freud and C. G. Jung.* Cambridge, MA: Harvard University Press, 1988.
Freud, S. (1909). Notes upon a case of obsessional neurosis. *S.E. 10.*
Freud, S. (1910). *Leonardo Da Vinci and a Memory of His Childhood. S.E. 11.*
Freud, S. (1911). Formulations on the two principles of mental functioning. *S.E. 12.*
Freud, S. (1915a). Observations on transference-love. *S.E. 12.*
Freud, S. (1915b). A case of paranoia running counter to the psycho-analytic theory of the disease. *S.E. 14.*
Freud, S. (1916–17). *Introductory Lectures on Psycho-Analysis. S.E. 16.*
Freud, S. (1920a). *Beyond the Pleasure Principle. S.E. 18.*
Freud, S. (1920b). The psychogenesis of a case of homosexuality in a woman. In *S.E. 18* (pp. 145–172).
Freud, S. (1921). *Group Psychology and the Analysis of the Ego. S.E. 14.*
Freud, S. (1923). *The Ego and the Id. S.E. 19.*
Freud, S. (1924). The loss of reality in neurosis and psychosis. *S.E. 19.*
Freud, S. (1926a). *Inhibitions, Symptoms and Anxiety. S.E. 20.*
Freud, S. (1926b). *The Question of Lay Analysis. S.E. 20.*
Freud, S. (1931). Female sexuality. *S.E. 21* (pp. 221–243).
Freud, S. (1933). *New Introductory Lectures on Psycho-Analysis. S.E. 22.*
Freud, S. (1950 [1895]). Project for a scientific psychology. *S.E. 1.*
Freud, S., & Weiss, E. (1920). *Problemas de la práctica psicoanalítica: Correspondencia Freud–Weiss.* Barcelona: Gedisa, 1979.
Friday, N. (1977). *My Mother/My Self: The Daughter's Search for Identity.* London: HarperCollins.
Friedman, J. A. (1998). *The Origins of Self and Identity: Living and Dying in Freud's Psychoanalysis.* Northvale, NJ: Jason Aronson.
Fryer, D. R. (2004). *The Intervention of the Other: Ethical Subjectivity in Levinas and Lacan.* New York: Other Press.

Gabel, J. (1962). *La Fausse conscience. Essai sur la reification*. Paris: Editions de Minuit.

Galenson, E. (1986). Early pathways to female sexuality in advantaged and disadvantaged girls. In T. Bernay & D. W. Cantor (Eds.), *The Psychology of Today's Women*. Hillsdale, NJ: Analytic Press.

Galenson, E., & Roiphe, H. (1976). Some suggested revisions concerning early female development. *Journal of the American Psychoanalytic Association, 5*: 29–57.

Gibeault, A. (2010). Introduction [to Section IV: Phantasy and representation]. In D. Birksted-Breen, S. Flanders & A. Gibeault (Eds.), *Reading French Psychoanalysis* (pp. 268–285). London: Routledge.

Ginsberg, A. (1956). *Howl and Other Poems*. San Francisco, CA: City Lights Books. Reprinted in *Collected Poems 1947–1985*. London: Penguin, 1995.

Ginzburg, C. (1989). *Clues, Myths, and the Historical Method*, trans. J. Tedeschi & A. C. Tedeschi. Baltimore, MD: Johns Hopkins University Press, 2013.

Gödel, K. (1931). Über formal unentscheidbare Sätze der *Principia Mathematica* und verwandter Systeme, 1. In S. Feferman (Ed.), *Kurt Gödel: Collected Works, Vol. 1* (pp. 144–195). Oxford: Oxford University Press, 1986.

Gomez, L. (2005). *The Freud Wars: An Introduction to the Philosophy of Psychoanalysis*. Hove: Routledge.

Green, A. (1980). Passions and their vicissitudes. On the relation between madness and psychosis. In *On Private Madness*. London: Hogarth Press, 1986.

Green, A. (2002). The central phobic position. In *Psychoanalysis: A Paradigm of Clinical Thinking*. London: Free Association Books, 2005. Reprinted as: The central phobic position: A new formulation of the free association method, in P. Williams (Ed.), *Key Papers on Borderline Disorders*. London: Karnac, 2005. And as: The central phobic position: With a model of the free-association method, in A. Green (Ed.), *Resonance of Suffering: Countertransference in Non-Neurotic Structures*. London: International Psychoanalytical Association, 2007; London: Karnac, 2009.

Grubrich-Simitis, I. (1995). *Early Freud and Late Freud: Reading Anew Studies on Hysteria and Moses and Monotheism*. London: Routledge, 1997.

Halberstadt-Freud, H. C. (1989). Electra in bondage. *Free Associations, 17*: 58–89.

Ham, C., & Berwick, D. (Eds.) (2017). *Organising Care at the NHS Front Line – Who Is Responsible?* London: The King's Fund. Available at www.kingsfund.org.uk/sites/default/files/field/field_publication_file/Organising_care_NHS_front_line_Kings_Fund_May_2017.pdf

Haslanger, S. (2017). Culture and critique. *Aristotelian Society Supplementary Volume, 91* (Issue 1, 1 June): 149–173.

Havighurst, C. C., Hutt, P. B., McNeil, B. J., & Miller, W. (2001). Evidence: Its meaning in health care and in law. *Journal of Health Politics, Policy and* Law, *26* (2): 195–216.

Hobson, R. P., & Kapur, R. (2005). Working in the transference: Clinical and research perspectives. *Psychology and Psychotherapy: Theory, Research and Practice, 78*: 275–293.

Hoffer, A. (1996). Asymmetry and mutuality in the analytic relationship: Contemporary lessons from the Freud–Ferenczi dialogue. In P. L. Rudnytsky, A. Bókay, & P. Giampieri-Deutsch (Eds.), *Ferenczi's Turn in Psychoanalysis*. New York: New York University Press.

Horney, K. (1924). On the genesis of the castration complex in women. *International Journal of Psychoanalysis, 5*: 50–65.

Horney, K. (1926). The flight from womanhood: The masculinity complex in women as viewed by men and by women. *International Journal of Psychoanalysis, 7*: 324–339.

Horney, K. (1932). The dread of woman: Observations on a specific difference in the dread felt by men and by women respectively for the opposite sex. *International Journal of Psychoanalysis, 13*: 348–360.

Horney, K. (1933). The denial of the vagina: A contribution to the problem of the genital anxieties specific to women. *International Journal of Psychoanalysis, 14*: 57–70.

Hoyningen-Huene, P. (1990). Kuhn's conception of incommensurability. *Studies in History and Philosophy of Science Part A, 21* (3): 481–492.

Isaacs, S. (1948). The nature and function of phantasy. *International Journal of Psychoanalysis, 29*: 73–97 Also in M. Klein, P. Heimann, S. Isaacs, & J. Riviere, *Developments in Psycho-Analysis*. London: Hogarth Press, 1952.

Jacobson, P. D. (2001). Cost-effectiveness analysis in the courts: Recent trends and future prospects. *Journal of Health Politics, Policy and Law, 26* (2): 291–326.

Jaques, E. (1955). Social systems as a defence against persecutory and depressive anxiety. In M. Klein, P. Heimann, & R. E. Money-Kyrle (Eds.), *New Directions in Psycho-Analysis*. London: Tavistock, 1971.

Joffe, W. G., & Sandler, J. (1979). Adaptation and individuation: An illustrative case. *Bulletin of the Anna Freud Centre, 2*: 127–161.

Jones, E. (1927). The early development of female sexuality. In *Papers on Psycho-Analysis* (pp. 438–451). London: Karnac, 1977.

Jones, E. (1933). The phallic phase. In *Papers on Psycho-Analysis* (pp. 452–484). London: Karnac, 1977.

Jones, E. (1935). Early female sexuality. In *Papers on Psycho-Analysis* (pp. 485–495). London: Karnac, 1977.

Kantor, I. L., Solodovnikov, A. S., & Shenitzer, A. (1989). *Hypercomplex Numbers: An Elementary Introduction to Algebras*. New York: Springer.

Karasu, T. B. (1986). The psychotherapies: Benefits and limitations. *American Journal of Psychotherapy, 40*: 324–343.
Kernberg, O. (2006). Research anxiety: A response to Roger Perron's comments. *International Journal of Psychoanalysis, 87* (4): 933–937.
Kerridge, R. K., & Saul, W. P. (2003). The medical emergency team, evidence-based medicine and ethics. *The Medical Journal of Australia, 179* (6): 313–315.
Khan, A., & Brown, W. A. (2015). Antidepressants versus placebo in major depression: An overview. *World Psychiatry, 14*: 294–300.
Khan, M. M. R. (1963). The concept of cumulative trauma. In *The Privacy of the Self*. London: Hogarth Press, 1974.
Klein, D. F., & Ross, D. C. (1993). National Institute of Mental Health Treatment of Depression Collaborative Research Program General Effectiveness Report. *Neuropsychopharmacology, 8*: 241–251.
Klein, M. (1926). The psychological principles of early analysis. *International Journal of Psychoanalysis, 8*: 25–37.
Klein, M. (1927). Symposium on child-analysis. *International Journal of Psychoanalysis, 8*: 339–370.
Klein, M. (1928). Early stages of the Oedipus complex. *International Journal of Psychoanalysis, 9*: 167–180, Reprinted in *The Writings of Melanie Klein, Vol. 1*. London: Hogarth Press/The Institute of Psycho-Analysis, 1975.
Klein, M. (1931). A contribution to the theory of intellectual inhibition. *International Journal of Psychoanalysis, 12*: 206–218.
Klein, M. (1932). The effects of early anxiety-situations on the sexual development of the girl. In *The Writings of Melanie Klein, Vol. 2*. London: Hogarth Press, 1975.
Klein, M. (1935). A contribution to the psychogenesis of manic-depressive states. *International Journal of Psychoanalysis, 16*: 145–174.
Klein, M. (1945). The Oedipus Complex in the light of early anxieties. *International Journal of Psychoanalysis, 26*: 11–33.
Klein, M. (1946). Notes on some schizoid mechanisms. In *The Writings of Melanie Klein, Vol. 3*. London: Hogarth Press.
Klein, M. (1957). Envy and gratitude. In *The Writings of Melanie Klein, Vol. 3*. London: Hogarth Press.
Klein, M., Heimann, P., Isaacs, S., & Riviere, J. (1952). *Developments in Psychoanalysis*. London: Hogarth Press.
Kohon, G. (1976). Nascita e morte nella schizophrenia. In A. Verdiglione (Ed.), *Il Diavolo sul lettino. Psicosi e follia*. Venezia: Marsilio, 1977.
Kohon, G. (1986). *The British School of Psychoanalysis: The Independent Tradition*. London: Free Association Books.
Kohon, G. (1999). *No Lost Certainties to Be Recovered*. London: Karnac.
Kohon, G. (2005). Love in the time of madness. In A. Green & G. Kohon, *Love and Its Vicissitudes*. London: Routledge.

Kohon, G. (2007). Borderline traces and the question of diagnosis. In A. Green (Ed.), *Resonance of Suffering: Countertransference in Non-Neurotic Structures*. London: International Psychoanalytical Association.
Kohon, G. (2016). *Reflections on the Aesthetic Experience: Psychoanalysis and the Uncanny*. London: Routledge/The Institute of Psychoanalysis.
Kohon, G. (2018). *British Psychoanalysis: New Perspectives in the Independent Tradition*. London: Routledge/The Institute of Psychoanalysis.
Kohon, G. (2019). Encountering the uncanny: Eduardo Chillida, Ai Weiwei, and the psychoanalytic frame. Paper presented at the Conference on The Uncanny: Art, Literature and the Clinic, The Institute of Psychoanalysis, London, 24 November. In C. Bronstein & C. Seulin (Eds.), *On Freud's "The Uncanny"* (in preparation).
Kristeva, J. (1983). *Tales of Love*. New York: Columbia University Press, 1987.
Kristeva, J. (2000). *Melanie Klein*. New York: Columbia University Press, 2001.
Kuhn, T. S. (1962). *The Structure of Scientific Revolutions* (3rd edition). Chicago, IL: University of Chicago Press, 1996.
Kuhn, T. S. (1987). What are scientific revolutions?. In J. Conant & J. Haugeland (Eds.), *The Road since Structure: Philosophical Essays, 1970–1993, with an Autobiographical Interview*. Chicago, IL: University of Chicago Press, 2000.
Lacan, J. (1936 [1949]). The mirror stage as formative of the function of the I. In *Ecrits: A Selection*. London: Tavistock, 1977.
Lacan, J. (1953). Some reflections on the ego. *International Journal of Psychoanalysis, 34*: 11–17.
Lacan, J. (1960–61). *Le Séminaire. Livre VIII. Le Transfert, 1960–61*, ed. J. A. Miller. Paris: Seuil, 1991.
Laing, R. D. (1960). *The Divided Self: An Existential Study in Sanity and Madness*. London: Tavistock.
Lampl-de Groot, J. (1927). The evolution of the Oedipus complex in women. In *The Development of the Mind*. London: Hogarth Press, 1966.
Laplanche, J. (1956). Implantation, intromission. In *Essays on Otherness*. Abingdon: Routledge, 1999.
Laplanche, J. (1987). *New Foundations for Psychoanalysis*. Oxford: Blackwell.
Laplanche, J., & Pontalis, J.-B. (1967). *The Language of Psychoanalysis*. London: Hogarth Press, 1973.
Lebovici, S. (1961). La relation objectale chez l'enfant. *Psichiatrie de L'Enfant, 3* (1): 147–226.
Leclaire, S. (1975). *Matan a un niño. Ensayo sobre el narcisismo primario y la pulsión de muerte*. Buenos Aires: Amorrortu Editores, 1977.
Lemma, A. (2014). The body of the analyst and the analytic setting: Reflections on the embodied setting and the symbiotic transference. *International Journal of Psychoanalysis, 95* (2): 225–244.

Levinas, E. (1975). *Sur Maurice Blanchot*. Montpellier: Fata Morgana.

Levinas, E. (1987). *Time and the Other and Additional Essays*. Pittsburgh, PA: Duquesne University Press.

Libbrecht, K. (1995). *Hysterical Psychosis: A Historical Survey*. New Brunswick, NJ: Transaction Publishers.

Little, M. (2003). "Better than numbers": A gentle critique of evidence-based medicine. *Australian and New Zealand Journal of Surgery*, *73*: 177–182.

Loewald, H. (1960). On the therapeutic action of psychoanalysis. *International Journal of Psychoanalysis*, *41*: 16–33.

Maleval, J.-C. (1981). *Folies hystériques et psychoses dissociatives*. Paris: Payot.

McDougall, J. (1964). Homosexuality in women. In J. Chasseguet-Smirgel (Ed.), *Female Sexuality*. London: Karnac, 1985.

McDougall, J. (1986). Eve's reflection: On the homosexual components of female sexuality. In H. C. Meyers (Ed.), *Between Analyst and Patient: Dimensions in Countertransference and Transference*. Hillsdale, NJ: Analytic Press.

Mijolla, A. de (1987). Unconscious identification fantasies and family prehistory. *International Journal of Psychoanalysis*, *58*: 397–403.

Miller, F. G., & Kaptchuk, T. J. (2008). The power of context: Reconceptualising the placebo effect. *Journal of the Royal Society of Medicine*, *101*: 222–225.

Minkowski, E. (1933). *Lived Time: Phenomenological and Psychopathological Studies*. Evanston, IL: Northwestern University Press, 1970.

Modell, A. H. (1990). *Other Times, Other Realities*. Cambridge, MA: Harvard University Press.

Money-Kyrle, R. (1956). Normal counter-transference and some of its deviations. *International Journal of Psychoanalysis*, *37*: 360–366. Reprinted in *The Collected Papers of Roger Money-Kyrle*. Strath Tay: Clunie Press, 1978.

Mulrow, C. D., & Cook, D. (Eds.) (1998). *Systematic Reviews: Synthesis of Best Evidence for Health Care Decisions*. Philadelphia, PA: American College of Physicians.

Mulrow, C. D., & Lohr, K. N. (2001). Proof and policy from medical research evidence. *Journal of Health Politics, Policy and Law*, *26* (2): 249–266.

Nabokov, V. (1948). Good readers and good writers. In F. Browers (Ed.), *Lectures on Literature*. Boston, MA: Houghton Mifflin Harcourt, 2003.

Neel, J. V., & Schull, W. J. (1954). *Human Heredity*. Chicago, IL: University of Chicago Press.

Ogden, T. (2005). *This Art of Psychoanalysis: Dreaming Undreamt Dreams and Interrupted Cries*. London: Routledge/The Institute of Psychoanalysis.

Patton, L. (Ed.) (2014). *Philosophy, Science, and History: A Guide and Reader*. New York: Routledge.

Peirce, C. S. (1903). *Collected Papers of Charles Sanders Peirce, Vol. 5*, ed. C. Hatshorne & P. Weiss. Cambridge, MA: Harvard University Press, 1958.

Perelberg, R. J. (1997). Introduction to Part I. In J. Raphael-Leff & R. J. Perelberg (Eds.), *Female Experience: Three Generations of British Women Psychoanalysts on Work with Women*. London: Routledge.

Perelberg, R. J. (2005). Introduction. In R. J. Perelberg (Ed.), *Freud: A Modern Reader* (pp. 14–19). London: Whurr.

Perelberg, R. J. (2007). Space and time in psychoanalytic listening. *International Journal of Psychoanalysis, 88* (6): 1473–1490.

Perelberg, R. J. (2015). On excess, trauma and helplessness: Repetitions and transformations. *International Journal of Psychoanalysis, 96* (6): 1453–1476.

Perelberg, R. J. (Ed.) (2018). *Psychic Bisexuality: A British–French Dialogue*. London: Routledge/The Institute of Psychoanalysis.

Piaget, J. (1973). The affective unconscious and the cognitive unconscious. *Journal of the American Psychoanalytic Association, 21*: 249–261.

Pichon-Rivière, E. J. (1947). Psicoanálisis de la esquizofrenia. *Revista Psiconanalítica, 4*: 614–618.

Pichon-Rivière, E. J. (1952). Quelques observations sur le transfert chez des patients psychotiques. *Revue Française de Psychanalyse, 16*: 254–258. Reprinted as: Algunas observaciones sobre la transferencia en pacientes psicóticos. *Revista de Psicoanálisis, 18* (No. 2, 1961).

Pichon-Rivière, E. J. (1965). *Lecciones de Psicología Social*. Course given at the Primera Escuela Privada de Psiquiatría. Buenos Aires.

Pichon-Rivière, E. J. (1967). Introducción a una nueva problemática de la psiquiatría. *Acta Psiquiátrica y Psicológica de América Latina, 13* (4): 355–365.

Pontalis, J.-B. (2000). *Windows*. Lincoln, NB: University of Nebraska Press, 2003.

Pritchett, J. (1993). *The Music of John Cage*. Cambridge: Press Syndicate of Cambridge University Press.

Qvortrup, L. (1998). *The Hypercomplex Society*. New York: Peter Lang, 2003.

Richardson, P., Kächele, H., & Renlund, C. (Eds.) (2004). *Research on Psychoanalytic Psychotherapy with Adults*. London: Karnac.

Riviere, J. (1958). A character trait of Freud's. In J. Sutherland (Ed.), *Psycho-Analysis and Contemporary Thought*. London: Hogarth Press. Reprinted in *The Inner World and Joan Riviere: Collected Papers 1920–1958*. London: Karnac, 1991.

Roiphe, H. & Galenson, E. (1981). *Infantile Origins of Sexual Identity*. New York: International Universities Press.

Rorty, R. (1989). *Contingency, Irony, and Solidarity*. Cambridge: Cambridge University Press.

Rorty, R. (1991). *Essays on Heidegger and Others: Philosophical Papers*. Cambridge: Cambridge University Press.

Rose, J., & Shulman, G. (Eds.) (2016). *The Non-Linear Mind: Psychoanalysis of Complexity in Psychic Life*. London: Karnac.

Rosenfeld, H. (1947). Analysis of a schizophrenic state with depersonalization. *International Journal of Psychoanalysis, 17*: 304–320, Reprinted in *Psychotic States: A Psychoanalytical Approach*. London: Hogarth Press, 1965; reprinted London: Karnac, 1982.

Rosenfeld, H. (1952). Notes on the psycho-analysis of the superego conflict in an acute schizophrenic patient. In *Psychotic States: A Psychoanalytical Approach*. London: Hogarth Press, 1965; reprinted London: Karnac, 1982.

Rosenfeld, H. (1983). Primitive object relations and mechanisms. *International Journal of Psychoanalysis, 64*: 261–267.

Rosenfeld, H. (1987). *Impasse and Interpretation: Therapeutic and Anti-therapeutic Factors in the Psychoanalytic Treatment of Psychotic, Borderline, and Neurotic Patients*. London: Tavistock.

Rost, F. (2018). Psychoanalysis needs research and research needs psychoanalysis. *New Associations, 25* (Summer): 8–9.

Rovelli, C. (2017). *The Order of Time*, trans. S. Carnell & E. Segre. London: Allen Lane, 2018.

Ruelle, D. (1980). Strange attractors. *Mathematical Intelligencer, 2*: 126–137.

Rustin, M. (1991). *The Good Society and the Inner World: Psychoanalysis, Politics and Culture*. London: Verso.

Rustin, M. (2001). *Reason and Unreason: Psychoanalysis, Science and Politics*. London: Continuum.

Sackett, D., & Guyau, II, G. (1992). Evidence-based medicine: A new approach to the teaching of medicine. *Journal of the American Medical Association, 268*: 2420–2425.

Santner, E. L. (2001). *On the Psychotheology of Everyday Life: Reflections on Freud and Rosenzweig*. Chicago, IL: University of Chicago Press.

Scott, D., & Usher, R. (Eds.) (1996). *Understanding Educational Research*. London: Routledge.

Segal, H. (1950). Some aspects of the analysis of a schizophrenic. In *The Work of Hanna Segal: A Kleinian Approach to Clinical Practice*. New York: Jason Aronson, 1981.

Segal, H. (1957). Notes on symbol formation. In *The Work of Hanna Segal: A Kleinian Approach to Clinical Practice*. New York: Jason Aronson, 1981.

Simms, B. R. (1986). *Music of the Twentieth Century: Style and Structure*. New York: Schirmer.

Slade, M., & Priebe, S. (Eds.) (2006). *Choosing Methods and Mental Health Research: Mental Health from Theory to Practice*. London: Routledge.

Somerville, C. & Morrison, V. (2018). Freeing up senior charge nurses' time through admin support. *Nursing Times, 114* (3): 27–29.

Spicer, A. (2018). *Business Bullshit*. London: Routledge.

Spillius, E. B. (2003). Anthropology and psychoanalysis: A personal concordance. *Bulletin of the British Psycho-Analytical Society, 39*: 7–24.

Stein, D. J. (2015). Antidepressant–placebo differences: Is the glass half full or half empty? [Editorial]. *World Psychiatry, 14* (3): 249–300.

Steiner, J. (1993). *Psychic Retreats: Pathological Organizations in Psychotic, Neurotic and Borderline Patients*. London: Routledge.

Steiner, J. (2013). Comments on the case of Raquel. *International Journal of Psychoanalysis, 94* (1): 99–104.

Stoller, R. (1976). Primary femininity. *Journal of the American Psychoanalytic Association, 24*: 59–78.

Székely, L. (1962). Symposium: The psycho-analytic study of thinking. *International Journal of Psychoanalysis, 43*: 297–305.

Tausk, V. (1919). On the origin of the "influencing machine" in schizophrenia. In R. Fliess (Ed.), *The Psycho-Analytic Reader: An Anthology of Essential Papers with Critical Introductions*. London: Hogarth Press, 1950.

Thompson, M. G. (1994). *The Truth about Freud's Technique: The Encounter with the Real*. New York: New York University Press.

Todorov, T. (1995). *Les Abus de la mémoire*. Paris: Arlea, 2015.

Tonelli, M. R. (2001). The limits of evidence-based medicine. *Respiratory Care, 46* (12): 1435–1440.

Torok, M. (1964). The significance of penis envy in women. In J. Chasseguet-Smirgel (Ed.), *Female Sexuality*. London: Karnac, 1985.

Tversky, A., & Kahneman, D. (1973). Availability: A heuristic for judging frequency and probability. *Cognitive Psychology, 2*: 207–232.

von Wietersheim, J., Malewski, P., Jäger, B., Köpp, W., Gitzinger, I., Köhler, P., et al. (2004). The German multi-centre eating disorder study on the influence of psychodynamic psychotherapy on personality. In P. Richardson, H. Kächele, & C. Renlund (Eds.), *Research on Psychoanalytic Psychotherapy with Adults*. London: Karnac.

Winnicott, D. W. (1945). Primitive early development. In *Collected Papers: Through Paediatrics to Psycho-Analysis*. London: Tavistock, 1958; reprinted London: Karnac, 1992.

Winnicott, D. W. (1947a). Further thoughts on babies as persons. In *The Child and the Outside World*. London: Tavistock, 1957.

Winnicott, D. W. (1947b). Hate in the counter-transference. In *Collected Papers: Through Paediatrics to Psycho-Analysis*. London: Tavistock, 1958; reprinted London: Karnac, 1992.

Winnicott, D. W. (1949 [1954]). Birth memories, birth trauma, and anxiety. In *Collected Papers: Through Paediatrics to Psycho-Analysis*. London: Tavistock, 1958; reprinted London: Karnac, 1992.

Winnicott, D. W. (1951). Transitional objects and transitional phenomena. In *Collected Papers: Through Paediatrics to Psycho-Analysis*. London: Tavistock, reprinted London: Karnac, 1992.

Winnicott, D. W. (1954). Metapsychological and clinical aspects of regression within the psycho-analytical set-up. In *Collected Papers: Through Paediatrics to Psycho-Analysis*. London: Tavistock, 1958; reprinted London: Karnac, 1992.

Winnicott, D. W. (1960a). Counter-transference. In *The Maturational Processes and the Facilitating Environment: Studies in the Theory of Emotional Development*. London: Hogarth Press/The Institute of Psycho-Analysis, 1965; London: Karnac, 1990.

Winnicott, D. W. (1960b). Ego distortion in terms of true and false self. In *The Maturational Processes and the Facilitating Environment: Studies in the Theory of Emotional Development*. London: Hogarth Press/The Institute of Psycho-Analysis, 1965; London: Karnac, 1990.

Winnicott, D. W. (1962). Ego integration in child development. In *The Maturational Processes and the Facilitating Environment: Studies in the Theory of Emotional Development*. London: Hogarth Press/The Institute of Psycho-Analysis, 1965; London: Karnac, 1990.

Winnicott, D. W. (1963 [1974]). Fear of breakdown. In *Psycho-Analytic Explorations*, ed. C. Winnicott, R. Shepherd & M. Davis. London: Karnac, 1989.

Winnicott, D. W. (1965). The psychology of madness: A contribution from psycho-analysis. In *Psycho-Analytic Explorations*, ed. C. Winnicott, R. Shepherd & M. Davis. London: Karnac, 1989.

Winnicott, D. W. (1968). Communication between infant and mother, and mother and infant, compared and contrasted. In W. G. Joffe (Ed.), *What Is Psychoanalysis?* London: Ballière, Tindall & Cassel/The Institute of Psycho-Analysis.

Winnicott, D. W. (1970). On the basis for self in body. In *Psycho-Analytic Explorations*, ed. C. Winnicott, R. Shepherd & M. Davis. London: Karnac, 1989.

Wollheim, R. (1984). *The Thread of Life: The William James Lectures 1982*. Cambridge: Cambridge University Press.

Žižek, S. (1997). *The Abyss of Freedom/Ages of the World*. Ann Arbor, MI: University of Michigan Press.

Žižek, S. (1998). Introduction: Cogito as a shibboleth. In S. Žižek (Ed.), *Cogito and the Unconscious*. Durham, NC: Duke University Press.

Index

Entries in notes are indicated by n.

For Product Safety Concerns and Information please contact our EU representative GPSR@taylorandfrancis.com
Taylor & Francis Verlag GmbH, Kaufingerstraße 24, 80331 München, Germany

www.ingramcontent.com/pod-product-compliance
Ingram Content Group UK Ltd.
Pitfield, Milton Keynes, MK11 3LW, UK
UKHW022314250926
475702UK00046B/783
9780367236502